Blood Groups

Edited by Anil Tombak

Published in London, United Kingdom

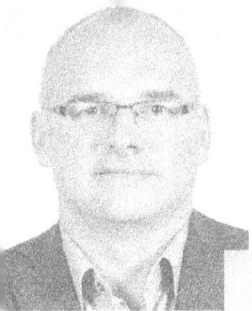
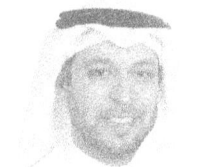
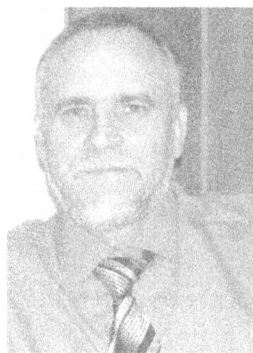
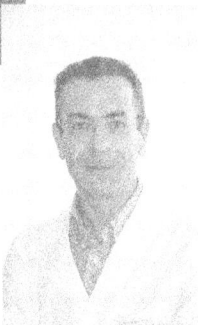
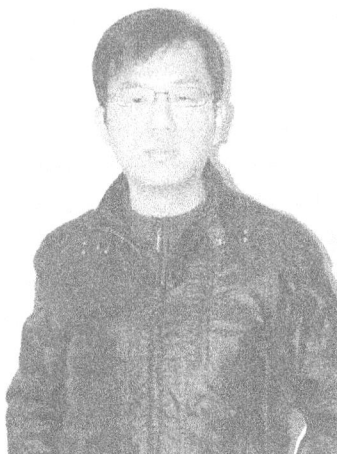
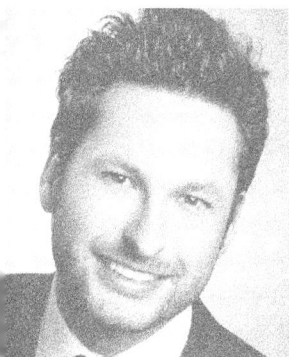
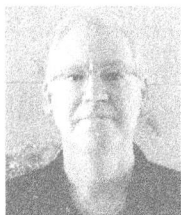

IntechOpen

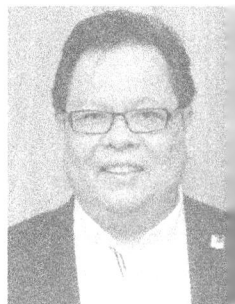
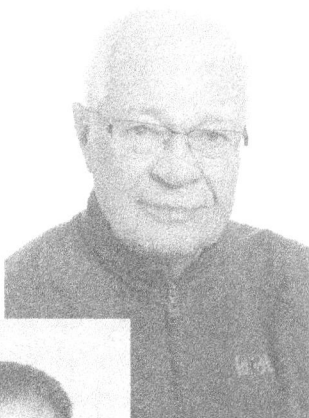
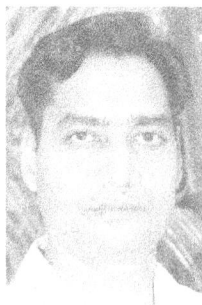
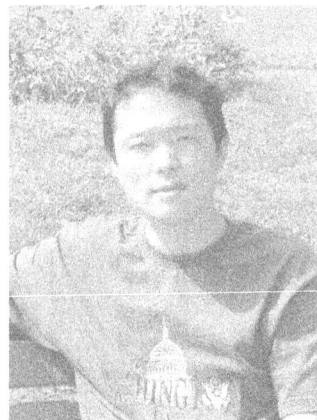
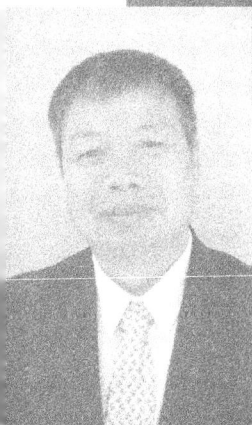
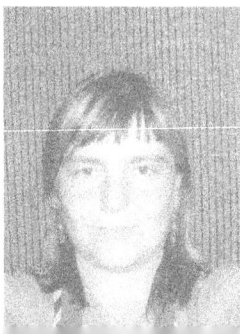

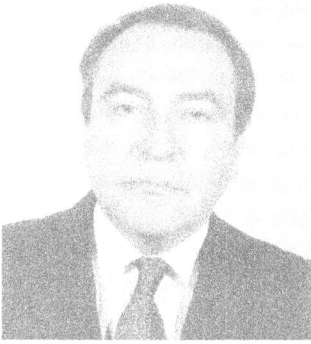

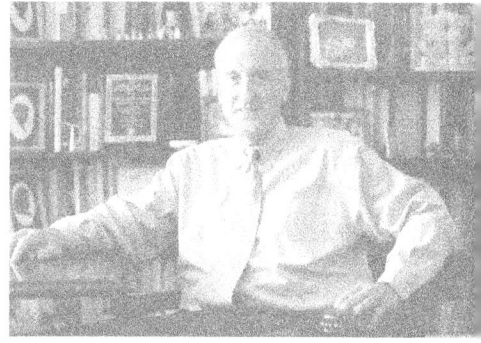

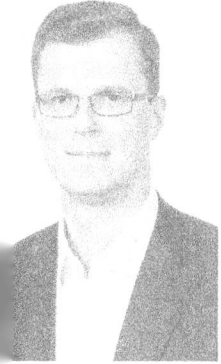

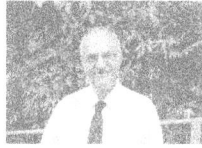

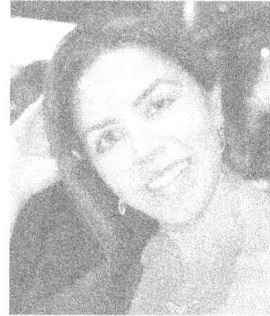

Supporting open minds since 2005

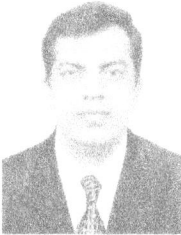

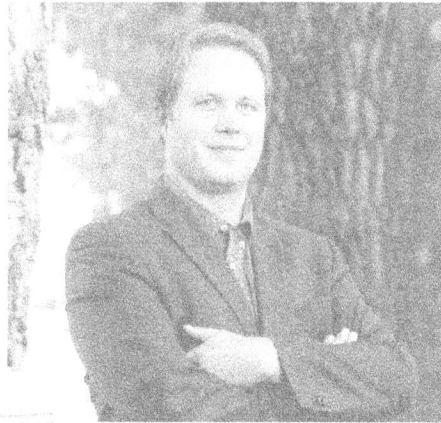

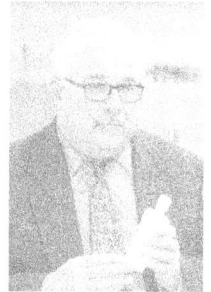

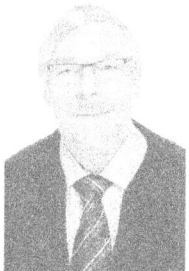

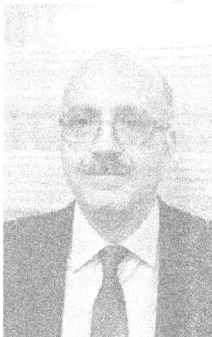

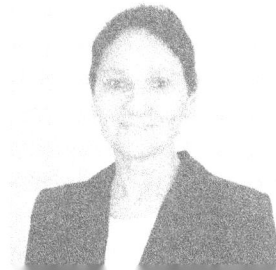

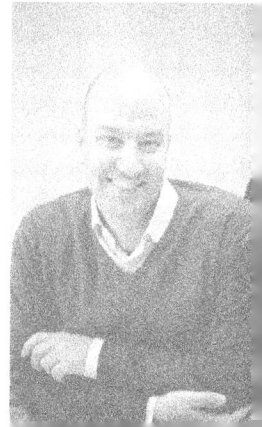

Blood Groups
http://dx.doi.org/10.5772/intechopen.73434
Edited by Anil Tombak

Contributors
Ebru Dündar Yenilmez, Soumya Das, Frida Gylmiyarova, Nataliya Kolotyeva, Valeriia Kuzmicheva, Oksana Gusyakova, Elena Ryskina, John Olaniyi, Anil Tombak

Notice
Statements and opinions expressed in the chapters are these of the individual contributors and not necessarily those of the editors or publisher. No responsibility is accepted for the accuracy of information contained in the published chapters. The publisher assumes no responsibility for any damage or injury to persons or property arising out of the use of any materials, instructions, methods or ideas contained in the book.

First published in London, United Kingdom, 2019 by IntechOpen
IntechOpen is the global imprint of INTECHOPEN LIMITED, registered in England and Wales, registration number: 11086078, The Shard, 25th floor, 32 London Bridge Street
London, SE19SG - United Kingdom
Printed in Croatia

British Library Cataloguing-in-Publication Data
A catalogue record for this book is available from the British Library

Additional hard and PDF copies can be obtained from orders@intechopen.com

Blood Groups
Edited by Anil Tombak
p. cm.
Print ISBN 978-1-83881-104-4
Online ISBN 978-1-83881-105-1
eBook (PDF) ISBN 978-1-83881-106-8

We are IntechOpen,
the world's leading publisher of
Open Access books
Built by scientists, for scientists

4,200+
Open access books available

116,000+
International authors and editors

125M+
Downloads

Our authors are among the

151
Countries delivered to

Top 1%
most cited scientists

12.2%
Contributors from top 500 universities

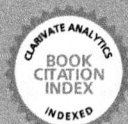

CLARIVATE ANALYTICS
BOOK
CITATION
INDEX
INDEXED

WEB OF SCIENCE™

Selection of our books indexed in the Book Citation Index
in Web of Science™ Core Collection (BKCI)

Interested in publishing with us?
Contact book.department@intechopen.com

Numbers displayed above are based on latest data collected.
For more information visit www.intechopen.com

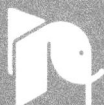

Meet the editor

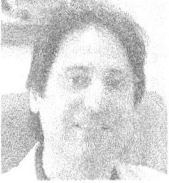

Assoc. Prof. Dr. Anil Tombak, MD, was born on April 25, 1976. He graduated from Gazi Anatolian High School in 1994 and then from Çukurova University Medical Faculty in 2000. Subsequently, he was trained at Mersin University Medical Faculty, Internal Medicine Department, and after internal medicine specialization, he became a Fellow of Hematology at the same University. He became a hematologist in 2013 and is still working at Mersin University Medical Faculty, Department of Internal Medicine-Hematology, Mersin, Turkey. He has performed research in several fields, with over 50 publications in (inter)national journals and numerous papers at scientific conferences. He received several awards and is a member of the Turkish Society of Hematology. Dr. Tombak is married and has two children.

Contents

Preface

Today, information in medical science is increasing rapidly, and with the communication age, accessing information is quite easy. However, with this increasing knowledge, information complexity has emerged. Thus, despite all this increasing knowledge, the interest and need for basic books have not diminished. Blood groups, erythrocyte antigens, and transfusion are fundamental areas of medicine and are related to many disciplines of science like hematology, immunology, surgery, and genetics. This book is a collection of current information related to blood groups and transfusion, and a practical resource for all concerned physicians.

I would like to thank all the authors and IntechOpen and hope that this book will be a stepping stone for scientists who are rapidly advancing their science journey.

Dr. Anil Tombak, MD
Associate Professor,
Department of Internal Medicine-Hematology,
Mersin University Medical Faculty,
Mersin, Turkey

Clinical Significance of Blood Groups

Chapter 1

Introductory Chapter: Blood Groups - From Past to the Future

Anil Tombak

1. Introduction

Because we know there are different blood groups today, doctors can save lives by transferring the right blood to patients. But previously, the blood transfusion was just a dream. This idea was first discussed by the doctors at the time of Renaissance. In later periods, a French doctor transfused calf blood to a patient in the 1600s and the patient died. Of course, blood transfusions which were made unaware of the presence of antigenic differences ended with death. Because of such unsuccessful trials, the blood transfusion gained a bad reputation. In 1817, Dr. James Blundell, an English obstetrician, said that living species had different blood structures, so blood could not be transfused between different species, but only human blood could be given to a human. In the following years, a total of 10 blood transfusions were performed, of which only 4 survived. Dr. Blundell did not know that human blood had different antigens, and people should be transfused with the same blood group antigens. And probably, this was the cause of death in some patients.

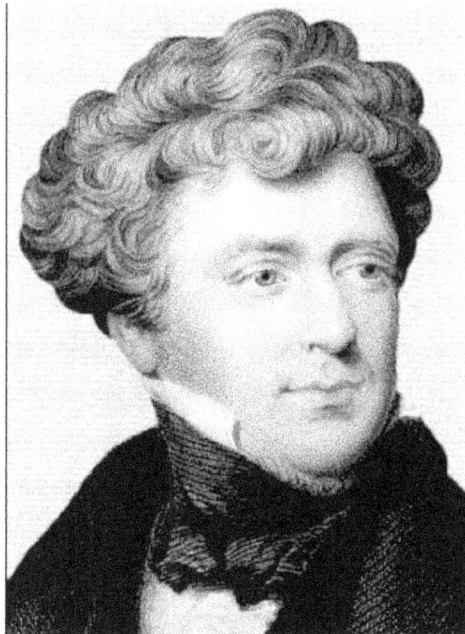

Dr. James Blundell

Karl Landsteiner identified ABO blood group antigens in 1900. And this was one of the most important steps in safe transfusion. He wondered what would happen when the bloods of healthy people mixed up and sometimes saw clots in healthy blood. When he separated the plasma with the red cells in the blood and mixed the plasma of the different bloods, he realized that clotting was involved in certain mixtures. He gave random names to these plasmas like A, B, and C. Later, C's name was changed to O; after a while, the AB group was found.

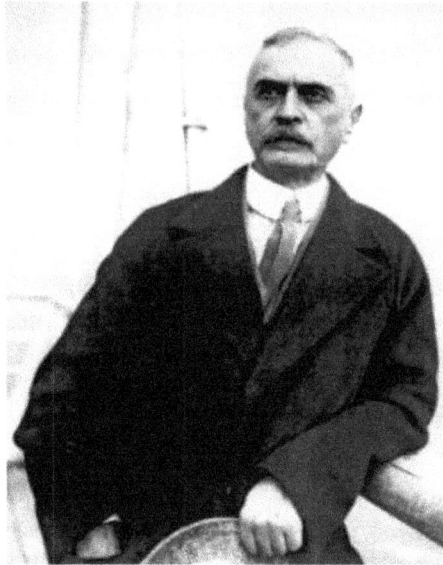

Dr. Karl Landsteiner

In the mid-twentieth century, American researcher Philip Levine discovered Rhesus (Rh) factor and classified the blood as Rh (+) and Rh (−).

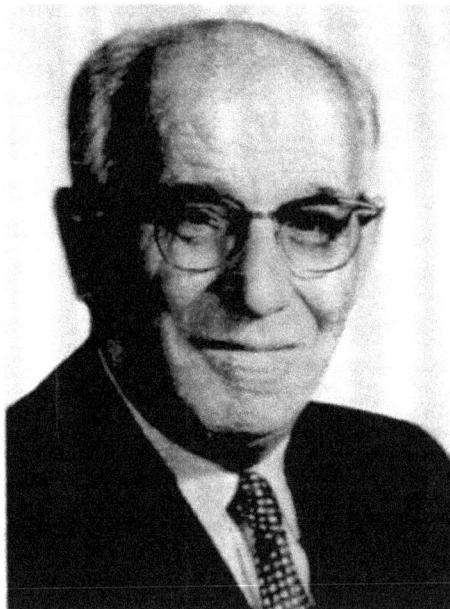

Dr. Philip Levine

In this still ongoing historical journey, today, blood groups are defined as hereditary characters on the surface of erythrocytes detected by a specific allo-antibody. International Society of Blood Transfusion (ISBT) reported that there are 33 blood group systems and more than 300 blood group antigens for these systems in humans. The structure of blood group antigens may be protein, glycoprotein, and glycolipid. The distribution of these antigens varies between people and societies, and between the human tissues, as well. Some of them are found just at the erythrocytes, at the other blood cells, and at the tissues. Blood groups are of great importance in transplantation, pregnancy, and transfusion. Some functions of blood group antigen are as follows: transport of some biological molecules toward the erythrocyte membrane, cell adhesion, autologous complement regulators, enzymes, receptors for external stimuli, anchors connecting the erythrocyte membrane to the cell skeleton, extracellular carbohydrates that protect the cell from the mechanical and microbial attacks, etc. Blood group antibodies may develop due to various reasons. These may be "natural antibodies" which develop in the first months of life as in ABO system or may be "immune antibodies" which develop due to transfusion, transplantation, or pregnancy. Antibodies against lots of erythrocyte antigens may cause severe transfusion reactions. For this reason, beside the tests where ABO and RhD antigen are evaluated, additional tests are needed to ensure transfusion safety. The goal is to maintain the vitality and the function of erythrocytes in the longest period and prevention of hemolysis after transfusion. For this purpose, to detect and type antibodies that may pose risk, we perform cross-match, antibody screening/identification, direct antiglobulin test and investigate minor blood group antigens.

2. Conclusion

Although the recent developments, the biological structure of most blood group antigens and their functions are still unknown, and we still have more ways to walk in this area. This book aims to reveal the latest developments related to "blood groups."

Author details

Anil Tombak
Mersin University, Mersin, Turkey

*Address all correspondence to: aniltombak@mersin.edu.tr

IntechOpen

Chapter 2

Blood Transfusion Reactions

John Ayodele Olaniyi

Abstract

Blood transfusion reaction/adverse transfusion reactions could be fatal/severe or mild, immediate or delayed, immunological or nonimmunological, and infectious or noninfectious, and attention is paid particularly to the incidence, possible causes and pathophysiology, clinical features, and management of each type with the aim of improving awareness and raising consciousness towards improving blood safety and judicious use of blood so as to forestall these blood transfusion reactions as much as possible. This chapter serves as a synopsis to adverse blood reactions, which are very common but apparently more often under-recognized and/or under-reported particularly in developing countries. This should sharpen the consciousness of all health practitioners involved in blood transfusion services towards taking measures at preventing transfusion reactions right from donor selection up to the infusion of blood into the recipients.

Keywords: adverse blood reactions, blood safety, judicious use of blood, clinical features, management, immunological, immediate, infectious

1. Introduction

Blood transfusion remains a life-saving therapy and according to World Health Organization (WHO) guidelines, of 10 units per 1000 population, approximately 8 million units of blood are currently needed to meet the transfusion demand for a population of about 800 million [1]. While in the industrialized world, blood provision and blood safety are well established, in Africa, there is limited access to blood, and provision of unsafe blood renders blood safety a major public health concern. Blood transfusion may be needed in circumstances like obstetric hemorrhage, road traffic accidents, armed conflicts, sickle cell disease, anaemias especially in children, malnutrition, HIV, malaria, and parasitic infections. It is therefore important to always highlight the blood transfusion reactions, possible causes, expected symptoms and signs, preventive measures, and appropriate management. This will further encourage judicious use of blood and blood components.

2. What is blood transfusion reaction?

Blood transfusion reaction refers to undesirable, unintended, adverse response to the administration of blood, blood components, or derivatives that are well thought-out to be definitely probable or possibly related to this product. About 0.5–3% of all transfusions result in transfusion reaction.

Blood transfusion reactions can basically be categorized as infectious or noninfectious. The majority of blood transfusion reactions are, nonetheless, noninfectious with outcomes ranging from nonsignificant consequences to death [2, 3]. However, the infectious effects are given more prominence than other adverse reactions.

For emphasis, when any unexpected or untoward symptom or sign occurs during or shortly after the transfusion of a blood component, a transfusion reaction must be considered as the precipitating event until confirmed otherwise [4].

3. Classification and incidence of adverse events

Broadly, BTR can be classified as infectious or noninfectious, immunological or nonimmunological, immediate or delayed, and mild or life threatening. The common, well known manifestations to all types of BTR include fever, chills, and urticaria [3, 5, 6] (**Table 1**).

3.1 The acute (life-threatening) BTRs

- Acute (immediate) haemolytic transfusion reaction

- Delayed haemolytic transfusion reaction

- Transfusion transmitted bacterial infection

- Anaphylaxis

- Transfusion-related acute lung injury (TRALI)

- Transfusion-associated circulatory overload (TACO)

3.1.1 Other acute noninfectious complications of blood transfusion

- Allergic reactions

- Anaphylaxis (IgA-deficient recipient)

- Lung damage from microaggregates (massive transfusion)

- Transfusion-associated circulatory overload ("TACO")

- Bacterial infection (mainly with platelet transfusion)

- Hypothermia (rapid infusion of refrigerated blood)

- Citrate toxicity/hypocalcemia (massive transfusion or apheresis)

- Graft-versus-host disease

- Air embolism

3.1.2 Classification of transfusion reactions based on immune or nonimmune

- Acute immunological (<24 hours)
  - Immediate (acute) haemolytic transfusion reaction
  - Febrile nonhemolytic.

- ○ Minor/major allergic.

- ○ Anaphylaxis.

- ○ TRALI.

- ○ Acute nonimmunological (<24 hours).

- ○ Bacterial contamination.

- ○ Transfusion-associated circulatory overload (TACO).

- • Delayed immunological (>24 hours).

- ○ Delayed haemolytic transfusion reaction.

- ○ Other delayed reactions.

- ○ Minor/major allergic.

- ○ Anaphylaxis.

- • Delayed nonimmunological (>24 hours).

- ○ Transfusion transmissible infections (TTIs) (HIV/HBV/HCV).

- ○ Transfusion-associated circulatory overload (TACO).

Tables 1, 3 and **5** refer to classification of BTRs.

Acute transfusion reactions	Delayed transfusion reactions
Acute haemolytic reaction (AHTR)	Delayed haemolytic reaction
Anaphylaxis	Transfusion transmitted infection
Bacterial contamination of blood component	Transfusion-associated graft-versus-host disease
Transfusion-associated acute long injury	Post-transfusion purpura
Transfusion-associated circulatory overload (TACO)	Iron overload
Allergic reaction	Immunosuppression
Febrile nonhemolytic transfusion reaction (FNHTR)	

Table 1.
Types of blood transfusion reactions.

Adverse events	Risk/unit
Mild allergic	1 in 100
FNH	1 in 300
TACO	1 in 700
TRALI	1 in 10,000
Bacteria contamination	1 in 10,000
Anaphylactic	1 in 40,000
Fatal haemolytic	1 in 1,000,000
HIV/HBV/HCV	1 in 1,000,000 to 8,000,000

Table 2.
Frequency of transfusion reactions.

3.2 Frequency of transfusion reactions

The risk per unit for each adverse event is as stated in **Table 2**.

4. Common signs and symptoms of blood transfusion

Although the signs and symptoms of BTR will be fully discussed under each type of blood transfusion reaction, it is important that these features be highlighted as it relates to each system.

- i. Circulatory: circulatory changes include changes in blood pressure, tachycardia, arrhythmia, bleeding, blood in urine, and increase in bleeding tendencies.

- ii. Pulmonary: pulmonary features include shortness of breath, dyspnea, wheezing, cough, and changes on chest X-ray.

- iii. Immune: itching, rash/hives, flushing, fever, and chills/rigors.

- iv. Others: Unexplained discomfort, back pain, chest pain, pain at the site of intravenous infusion and along the course of the vein, and anxiety.

4.1 Recognition at bedside

The complex background clinical condition of critically ill patients could mask the symptoms of a serious blood transfusion reaction; therefore, ventilated patients could have increased peak airway pressures, hyperthermia, and changes in urine output or color in the context of a blood transfusion, during a massive transfusion protocol. Therefore, monitoring core temperature, prompt use of measures to avoid hypothermia, using blood warmers, watch for hypocalcaemia, acidosis, and hyperkalemia go a long way in unmasking blood transfusion reactions.

5. Types of transfusion reactions

5.1 Minor transfusion reaction symptoms

A BTR is regarded as minor if:

- The hives or rash cover less than 25% of the body and there are no other symptoms.

- The fever (1°C rise over baseline and higher than 38°C) is associated with no other symptoms.

Quick steps to take when temperature increases by >1°C and >38°C (**Table 3**)

- Stop transfusion

- Clerical check

- Notify physician

- Notify blood bank

If clerical error is established or additional serious symptoms are identified, do not order for restart of blood transfusion. Instead

- Administer acetaminophen 325 mg

- Continue to monitor patient carefully and frequently

- Stop transfusion if symptoms worsen or additional symptoms develop

- If uneventful, complete transfusion reaction investigation form

- Send to blood bank with blood sample as per algorithm

 Suspect

- Hemolytic transfusion reaction

- Bacterial contamination

Initiate transfusion reaction if the abovementioned points are excluded in investigation by

- Completing form 3.

- Collecting blood samples

- Sending blood bag to blood bank

- Continuing to monitor patient

- Reporting the condition to physician

The predominant symptom of a fever is most commonly seen in:

- Acute hemolytic transfusion reactions (AHTR)

- Febrile nonhemolytic transfusion reactions (FNHTR)

- Bacterial sepsis or contamination

5.2 Febrile nonhemolytic transfusion reaction (FNHTR)

The incidence of FNHTR is 1 in 300 for RBC concentrate transfusion and 1 in 20 for platelet concentrate transfusion.

Pathophysiological FNHTRs develop in patients that already have anti-leukocyte antibodies. Anti-leukocyte antibodies are raised in multiply transfused patients and multiparous women usually following RBC or platelet transfusions. In addition, donor-derived leukocytes present in platelets and RBC products liberate cytokines in the course of storage of blood and may also mediate NHTRs. Such cytokines include IL1, IL6, IL8, and TNF. Therefore, pre-storage leukoreduction may reduce the accumulation of these biologic mediators and the incidence of febrile, hypotensive, or hypoxic transfusion reactions.

Check for haemolysis	

Check for haemolysis
Perform visual examination of patient's plasma and urine (plasma and urine hemoglobin can be checked but this is not essential).
Blood film may show spherocytosis.
Bilirubin and lactate dehydrogenase (LDH) levels will be raised.

Check for incompatibility
Check the documentation and the patient's identity.
Repeat ABO group of patient pre-transfusion and post-transfusion and of the donor unit(s).
Screen the patient for red cell antibodies pre-transfusion and post-transfusion
Repeat crossmatch with pre-transfusion and post-transfusion samples.
Direct antiglobulin test (DAT) on pre- and post-transfusion samples.
Eluate from patient's red cells.

Check for disseminated intravascular coagulation
Perform blood count and film, coagulation screen, and fibrin degradation products (or D-dimers).

Check for renal dysfunction
Check blood urea, creatinine, and electrolytes.

Check for bacterial infection
Take blood cultures from the patient and donor unit including immediate Gram stain.

Immunological investigations
Check immunoglobulin A (IgA) levels and anti-IgA antibodies.

Table 3.
Investigations indicated in transfusion reactions.

Clinical presentation: fever during transfusion or up to 4 hours after. The patient may also experience chills, rigors, nausea and vomiting, and hypotension without fever. FNHTRs typically manifest during or within 4 hours of transfusion with fever (defined as an increase in temperature of 1°C above the patient's baseline temperature, typically to 38°C) with or without chills and/or rigors. Such reactions may also manifest primarily with chills and/or rigors with minimal or absent febrile component particularly in patients receiving antipyretics. Symptoms are self-limited and respond to symptomatic treatment, which includes antipyretics for fever and chills and meperidine for rigors. Close differentials to FNHTRs include acute haemolytic transfusion reaction and septic transfusion reactions and patients' underlying medical condition. Therefore, it is important to do necessary investigations to rule out haemolysis. Leukoreduction has been associated with significant reduction in FNHTRs.

Management: blood transfusion should be stopped immediately and the ordering physician should be informed. Blood transfusion may be restarted cautiously as directed after the thorough investigation (**Table 3** and **Algorithm 1**).

5.3 Acute haemolytic transfusion reaction (AHTR)

The incidence of AHTR is 1 in 38,000. It is caused by transfusion of incompatible ABO blood group to a patient. It can be fatal with a mortality rate of about 10% and the risk of death is directly proportional to the amount of incompatible blood transfused.

Clinical presentation: fever and chills happen to be the most common feature. Anxiety, pain at the site of infusion, nausea/vomiting, back pain, dyspnea, flushing, wheezing and passage of red color urine, haemoglobinuria, hypotension, renal failure, disseminated intravascular coagulation (DIC), and shock may occur as late/terminal complications.

Suspected acute transfusion reaction

- STOP transfusion
- IV open
- CONFIRM correct product for patient
- ASSESS patient for fever, cardiovascular status, respiratory status, urticaria/angioedema

No fever, Respiratory distress	Fever +/- chills, Respiratory distress, Hypotension	Fever/chills, Otherwise asymptomatic	Fever +/- chills, Hypotension, Flank/back pain, Bleeding	Fever +/- chills, +/- Hypotension	Urticaria/pruritus, Bronchospasm, Angioedema, Hypotension
TACO suspected	TRALI suspected	FNHTR suspected	AHTR suspected	Sepsis suspected	Urticarial or anaphylactic reaction suspected

Chest radiography, oxygenation status (TACO, TRALI)

- DAT (Coombs) test
- CBC, urine dipstick (AHTR)

Supportive data:	Supportive data:	Supportive data:	Supportive data:	Supportive data:	Supportive data:
Hypoxia; Infiltrate on CXR; Diuretic response; Hypertension; High cardiac filling pressures; High NT-proBNP; Cardiac history; Older age; Large infusion volume	Hypoxia; Infiltrate on CXR; Pink frothy airway secretions; Transient leukopenia; Onset during or within six hours of transfusion	Lack of any findings associated with AHTR, TRALI, sepsis, or other systemic illness (ie, diagnosis of exclusion); Non-leukoreduced blood products	Hemoglobinemia; Hemoglobinuria; Positive DAT; Low haptoglobin; High LDH; bilirubin; Findings of DIC; Clerical error discovered	Positive gram stain and culture; Visibly cloudy product or precipitate; More common with platelets. Infection may also be related to the patient underlying illness	Urticarial reactions have urticaria alone; Anaphylactic reactions may have: Wheezing, Angioedema, Hypotension, Low IgA level; anti-IgA

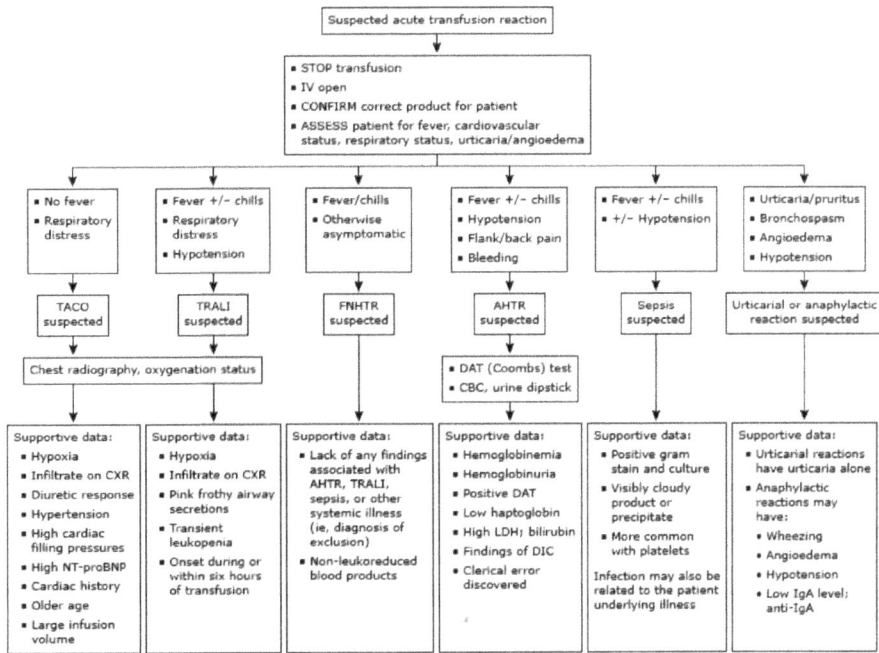

Algorithm 1.
Algorithm to follow in investigating acute transfusion reaction.

Pathophysiology: the ABO isohemagglutinins are compliment fixing and lead to intravascular destruction of transfused red cells which can manifest as hemoglobinemia and haemoglobinuria. Often, fever is the only initial sign. Activation of compliments leads to the release of cytokines like tumor necrosis factor, which is responsible for the fever and chills. The serologic hallmark of acute haemolytic reaction is a positive direct antiglobulin test (DAT), which demonstrates both IgG and compliment on the surface of recipient circulating red cells. Disseminated intravascular coagulation also occurs and bleeding may result.

Possible sources of error/causes include patient misidentification due to clerical error or failure to follow established hospital procedures. Therefore, definitive bedside patient identification, both at the time type and screening specimen, is being obtained, and the time the product is to be administered is very crucial. It has been advocated that the risk of mistransfusion can be greatly reduced by using barcode and radiofrequency chip technologies in order to ensure correct patient identification.

Also, AHTR can occur after platelet transfusions, typically involving a group A patient receiving group O platelets that contain high titer anti-A antibody.

Management: the treatment of AHTR is mainly supportive and it includes taking the following steps:

- STOP the transfusion!

- Check if any clerical errors in identifying the patient, blood group, and product label

- Notify the practitioner and blood bank, return product, and recollect sample from patient to confirm blood group

- Monitor patient closely

- Institute fluids and vaso-pressures for hypotension and urinary output.

5.4 Bacterial sepsis or contamination

The incidence of bacterial contamination for RBC is 1 in 50,000, 1 in 250,000 symptomatic septic reactions, and 1 in 500,000 with fatal bacterial sepsis. The incidence of bacterial contamination for platelet is 1 in 1000 with 1 in 10,000 symptomatic septic reactions and 1 in 60,000 fatal bacterial sepsis. About 10% of transfusion-related deaths are associated with bacterial sepsis.

Clinical presentation: the clinical features are similar to that of AHTRs and comprises of chills, rigors, high grade fever, tachycardia, hypotension, nausea, and vomiting. Disseminated intravascular coagulation (DIC) and shock may occur. Close examination of blood bag may reveal clots and change in color of blood in the bag compared to blood in the segmented tubing. There is no obvious focus of infection in the patient. The reaction typically develops 9–24 hours post transfusion and usually in neutropenic patients.

Management: such blood transfusion should be discontinued, if suspected and a doctor should be notified immediately who will notify and return the product to the blood bank after careful documentation of events. Necessary investigations should be carried out notably and blood culture samples should be collected. All necessary supportive interventions should be applied as dictated by the patient's clinical condition and the patient should be closely monitored. Also, abnormal bleeding or oozing in a patient during surgery that is equally having blood transfusion may raise suspicion of acute haemolytic transfusion reaction with DIC and appropriate management should be promptly applied (**Algorithm 2**).

5.5 Delayed haemolytic transfusion reaction (DHTRs)

In DHTRs, the patients develop an alloantibody to an RBC antigen following previous transfusion, pregnancy, or HSCT. Such red blood cell alloantibodies may decrease in titer although remaining clinically important, and hence, the patient has apparently negative antibody screening because the titer of the antibody has fallen below the detectable limit. In the event of a subsequent transfusion, the patient develops an anamnestic immune response to the mismatched antigen leading to delayed antibody-mediated destruction of transfused RBCs.

Clinical manifestation of AHTRs occurs 5–15 days post transfusion and it comprises haemoglobinuria, jaundice, and pallor as a result of the acute haemolytic process. In the context of a sickle cell disease patient (SCD) that often receives blood transfusion because of hyper-haemolytic crises, these features of haemolytic transfusion reaction are often accompanied by features of vaso-occlusive crisis (VOC), that is, pain, fever, and acute chest syndrome. There is usually worsened anemia and reticulocytopenia. In fact, DHTR is often misdiagnosed as VOC in SCD patient and the patient is unduly further transfused which culminates in multi-organ failure [5–9].

When features of AHTRs manifest, the link to the preceding transfusion is not always obvious. Direct antiglobulin test (DAT) is often positive for IgG, with or without compliment, depending on the antibody if carried out at this point. Also, an eluate may be performed to remove the IgG coating the circulating RBCs in order to identify it because a positive DAT may be unspecific. The antibody screen may also demonstrate the presence of a new antibody, although this may lag behind a positive DAT by a few days. The haemolysis in DHTRs is IgG mediated and thus extravascular; however, it is noteworthy that alloantibodies to Kidd blood group

1. STOP THE TRANSFUSION IMMEDIATELY and keep the IV line open with 0.9% saline
2. Contact the physician/authorized practitioner for medical assessment and document name of physician/authorized practitioner notified
3. Check vital signs at least every 15minute until stable
4. Check all labels, tags, treatment order, forms and the patient's identification band to determine if there is a clerical discrepancy
5. Notify the blood bank/lab

PHYSICIAN/AUTHORIZED PRACTITIONER WILL DETERMINE IF TRANSFUSION SHOULD CONTINUE
NOTE: REACTIONS IN A PATIENT TRANSFUSED FOR THE FIRST TIME MAY BE POTENTIALLY MORE SERIOUS

Serious Signs and Symptoms? **Clerical Discrepancy?**

IF THE PATIENT DEVELOPS ANY ONE OR MORE OF THE FOLLOWING DURING TRANSFUSION:
- Hypotension/shock
- Nausea/vomiting
- Rigors
- Hemoglobinuria
- Anxiety
- Febrile and 1°C rise over baseline
- Back/chest pain
- Tachycardia/arrhythmia

- DO NOT RESTART THE TRANSFUSION
- Institute patient management
- Send the following to the Blood Bank/Lab IMMEDIATELY:
  - Adults: 10-12mL of blood in EDTA tubes
  - Pediatrics: 3mL of blood in an EDTA tube
  - Completed Transfusion Reaction Investigation Form (CM105)
  - Blood and blood component and administration set/fluid
- consider
  - Blood and blood component cultures if patient temperature is ≥38°C

Serious Transfusion Reactions:
- Serious Febrile Non-Hemolytic
- Acute Hemolytic
- Anaphylactic
- Severe Allergic
- Fluid Overload
- Bacterial Contamination

- On physician/authorized practitioner direction:
  - Treat with Diphenhydramine 25-50 mg IV or PO (pediatric 0.5-1.0mg/Kg IV or PO to a maximum of 50 mg)
- Remain with patient and **observe** for the first 15 minutes after resuming

- On physician / authorized practitioner direction:
  - Treat with Acetaminophen 650mg PO or PR (pediatric 10-15mg/Kg PO)
- Resume transfusion cautiously
- Remain with patient and observe for the first 15 minutes after

If remainder of transfusion is uneventful, send to Blood Bank/Lab as soon as possible:
- A completed Transfusion Reaction Investigation Form (CM105)
- Blood specimens not required

IMMEDIATELY Stop the transfusion if patient develops any Serious Signs and Symstoms, follow serious signs and symptoms

If remainder of transfusion is uneventful, send to Blood Bank/Lab IMMEDIATELY:
- A completed Transfusion Reaction Investigation Form (CM105)
  - Adults: 10-12mL of blood in EDTA tubes
  - Pediatrics: 3mL of blood in an EDTA tube

Minor Allergic Reaction

Minor Febrile Non-

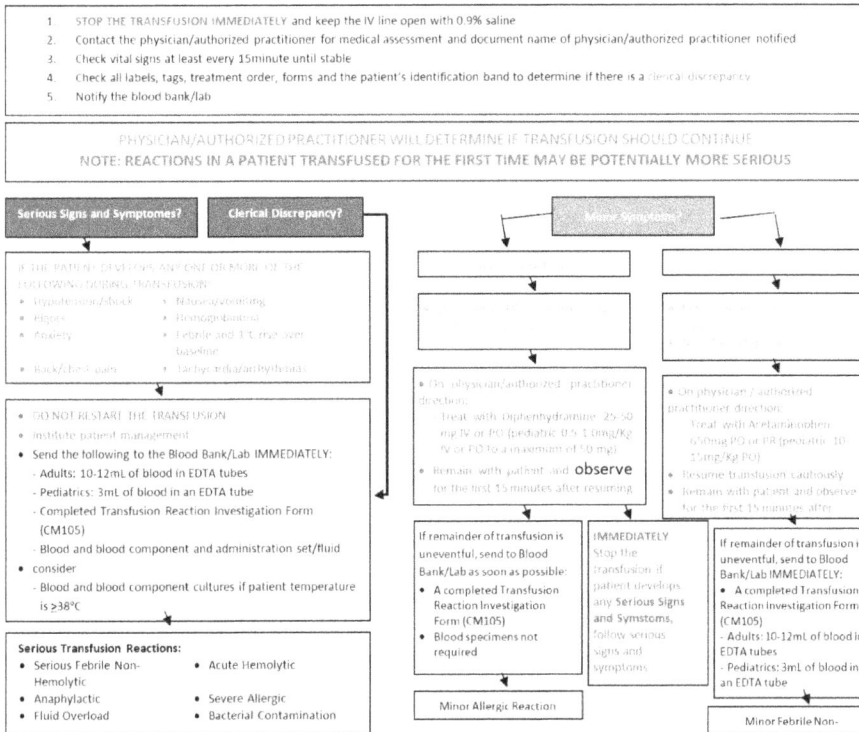

Algorithm 2.
Necessary steps in the management of blood transfusion reactions.

antigens may fix compliment and cause intravascular haemolysis with consequent haemoglobinuria, and occasional instances of severe complications like acute renal failure or disseminated intravascular coagulation have been reported. The antibodies most often implicated in DHTRs are directed against antigens in the Rh (34%), Kidd (30%), Duffy (14%), Kell (13%), and MNSs (4%) [8, 10]

5.5.1 Management of DHTRs

Ensure leukocyte-poor products as a preventive measure (refer **Algorithm 2**).

5.6 Transfusion-related acute lung injury (TRALI)

A consensus definition of TRALI is acute lung injury (ALL) occurring during a transfusion or within 6 hours of completing a transfusion with no other temporarily associated causes of acute lung injury (ALL). ALL is defined as (i) a syndrome of 10 acute onsets, (ii) hypoxemia ($PaO_2/FiO_2 < 300$ mm of Hg, O_2 saturation < 90% on room air or other clinical evidence), (iii) bilateral pulmonary infiltrates, and (iv) no evidence of circulatory overload [7, 11].

The development of TRALI, which is a potentially life-threatening reaction, is triggered by passive transfusion of donor anti-granulocyte antibodies (anti-HLA or anti HNA antibodies), cytokines, biologically active lipids, or other substances into the recipient. These cause acute lung injury with noncardiogenic pulmonary edema. The signs and symptoms comprise dyspnea, hypoxemia, hypotension, fever, and a chest X-ray showing bilateral lung infiltrates with pulmonary edema (**Figure 1**) [7, 11].

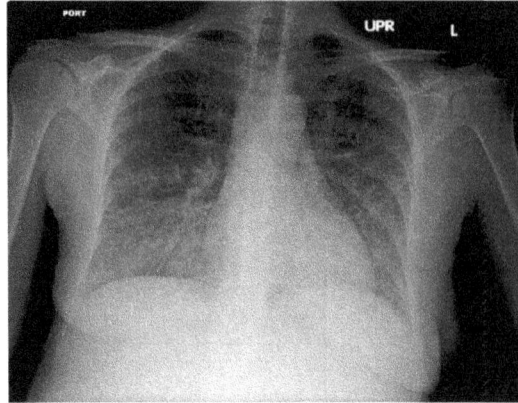

Figure 1.
CXR of a TRALI patient showing pulmonary infiltrates.

Management: aggressive pulmonary support including mechanical ventilation is frequently required. Approximately 80% of patients improve within 48–96 hours and all the patients require oxygen support with approximately 70% needing mechanical ventilation. Infrequently, antibodies in the recipient may react with donor granulocytes that were present in units of RBCs or platelets transfused. Strangely, in some cases of TRALI, neither recipient nor donor-derived antibodies can be identified. Other mechanisms have been advanced such as the priming of neutrophils by bioactive lipids that accumulate during blood storage (**Figure 2**) [7, 11].

The United States FDA in 2007 documented that TRALI represented 65% of all transfusion-related fatalities. The widespread implementation of TRALI risk reduction strategies adopted thereafter led to reduction to 37% of transfusion fatalities reported in the 5-year period from 2008 to 2012. TRALI remains the leading cause of death due to transfusion in the US.

The probable incidence rate of TRALI is about 1/5000 transfusions of plasma containing blood product, that is, RBCs, platelets, concentrate, platelet apheresis units, and plasma with a 5–10% fatality rate. TRALI may be difficult to differentiate from manifestations of patients underlying medical problems particularly those of cardiac origin, such as congestive heart failure and fluid overload brought on by transfusion.

Clinical management is supportive with the goal of reversing progressive hypoxemia. There is no universal method to prevent TRALI. Once blood from a particular patient is implicated in a case of TRALI, the donor is excluded from the donor pool. Preventing the first case of TRALI by those donors, however, requires the elimination of all blood donors whose plasma contain anti-HLA or anti-neutrophil antibodies. For plasma, this is achieved by excluding female donors from the plasma donor pool because multiparous females are most likely among a healthy donor population to have anti-HLA antibodies as a result of sensitization during pregnancy [7, 11]

When this approach was adopted in the UK in late 2003, where 60% of TRALI had been caused by plasma transfusions, no report of TRALI death due to plasma occurred after 2004 (6 deaths occurred in 2005, none from plasma). Major blood suppliers in the US now limit the use of female plasma or screen for HLA or HNA antibodies in multiparous donors. Even with these precautions in place, cases of TRALI in which HLA or any other granulocyte-specific antibodies do not appear to be responsible will not be eliminated.

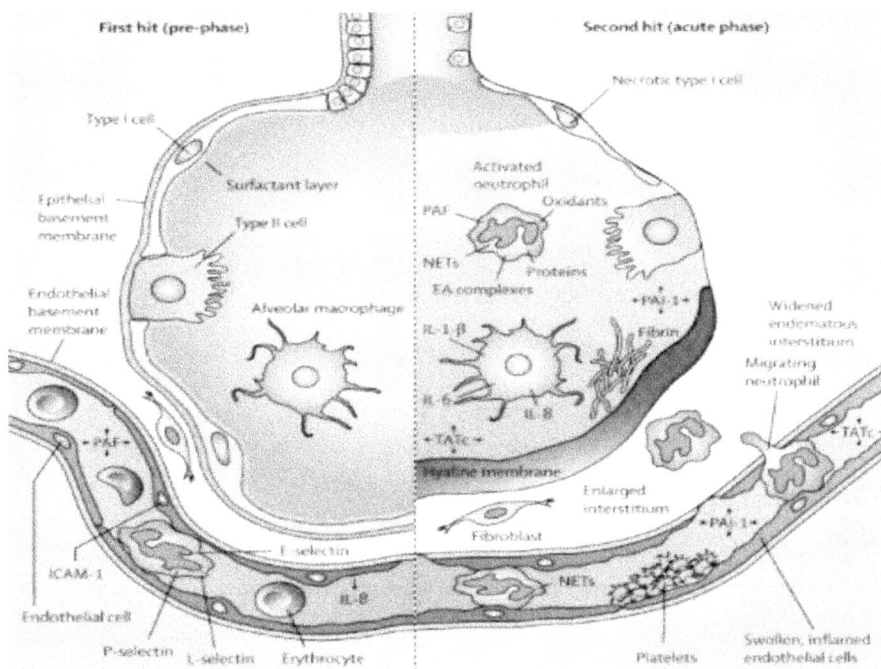

Figure 2.
Pathophysiologic mechanisms in TRALI. This figure illustrates inflammatory processes in the lung both during the "first hit" and during the "second hit" (acute phase) where the inflammatory processes are heightened than the "first hit". Mediators of inflammation in the infused blood products (FFP > platelets > RBCs) containing donor anti-granulocyte antibodies (anti-HLA and anti-HNA antibodies) along with cytokines and biologically active lipids activate inflammatory cascade through polymorph-nuclear cells (PMNs) with resultant capillary injury. As shown in the "second hit" section of the lung, the capillaries are congested, endothelial cells are swollen and inflamed, and there is increased platelet deposition and aggregation. The interstitial becomes more enlarged. There is increased adherence and migration of neutrophils of activated adhesion molecules (ICAM-1, P-Selectin, L-Selectin). Also, alveolar macrophages liberate inflammatory cytokines (IL-1b, IL-6, IL-8) and activated neutrophils elaborate PAF, NET compliments, and oxidant proteins. All these culminated in lung injury with noncardiogenic pulmonary edema causing hypoxemia, hypotension, pulmonary infiltrates, and fever.

Therefore, strict transfusion criteria for plasma-rich blood products, early recognition, and prompt clinical management are the keys to dealing with these potentially fatal transfusion reactions.

Reporting suspected cases of TRALI to the blood bank is also important in limiting potential risk to other patients by quarantine of any co-components from the same donation and evaluating the donor with possible exclusion from future donation if TRALI is confirmed [7, 11].

5.7 Transfusion-associated circulatory overload (TACO)

The incidence of TACO is 1/100 and the risk factors in TACO include patients with limited cardiopulmonary reserve, that is, the very young and the very old, high volume transfusion, background renal, or cardiac disease.

The onset is usually 1–2 hours post transfusion. TACO manifests as shortness of breath, cough, chest tightness, cyanosis, rales, orthopnea tachycardia, distended jugular veins, S3 gallop, and pulmonary edema, which are consistent with cardiac decompensation following volume overload [7, 12].

It is important that the vital signs of a patient under general anesthesia and on blood transfusion be continually monitored in order to be able to detect these features early and to be able to prevent TACO.

Managing

- Stop transfusion

- Position patient in upright position

- Supplementary oxygen

- Diuretics

- Cardiac and respiratory support as required

- Initiate transfusion reaction investigation

However, it is important to bear in mind the differences between TACO and TRALI (**Table 4**).

5.8 Allergic transfusion reactions

Allergic reactions following blood transfusions can be mild and frequently manifested by urticarial rash. Many urticarial reactions are donor-specific and thus do not occur with subsequent transfusion.

5.8.1 Management

If a recipient experiences multiple urticarial reactions, premedication with anti-histamines should be considered.

Washed products re-suspended in albumin or saline may be considered in severe cases. While removing plasma through washing mitigates allergic reactions, washing platelets impair platelet functions and lead to accelerated clearance after transfusion.

Antihistamines generally alleviate symptoms of allergic reactions but have not been proven to prevent them [7, 13].

5.8.2 Anaphylactic reaction

The incidence of anaphylactic reaction is put at 1 in 40,000 and the clinical presentation is characterized by widespread rash, shortness of breath cough, tachycardia, flushing, and anxiety.

	TRALI	TACO
Blood pressure	Low-normal	Normal-high
Body temperature	Normal-elevated	Normal
CXR	No vascular congestion	Vascular congestion, pleural effusion
BNP	Low (< 250 pg/ml)	High
PAOP	Low-normal	High
Ejection fraction	Normal function	Abnormal function
Response to diuretics	Inconsistent	Improved
Edema fluid	Transudate	Exudate

Table 4.
Differences between TRALI and TACO.

Severe IgA-deficient patients may make anti IgA antibody that can cause anaphylactic reaction, but this is a rare occurrence. Considering that approximately 1 in 1200 people is IgA deficient with anti-IgA antibodies and that passively transfused anti IgA antibodies do not cause allergic reactions, the pathophysiology of recurrent and severe allergic transfusion reactions in IgA deficiency is incompletely understood. Washed RBCs, washed platelets, and/or platelet and plasma products from IgA-deficient donors should be transfused only when a patient has severe IgA deficiency and a concern for anaphylactic reactions. Most IgA-deficient patients, even those with anti IgA, have no adverse reactions to transfusion. There are also reports of patients with deficiency of haptoglobin and various complement components such as C4a (Rogers antigen) or C4b (Chido antigen) developing anaphylactic reactions to platelets [7, 13].

Management: as illustrated in **Table 5** and **Algorithm 1**.

If hives/rash covers <25% of body stop transfusion; do the following: clerical check, notify physician, and notify blood bank.

If clerical error is identified or there are serious symptoms do not restart transfusion, the following should be ensured:

1. Administer diphenhydramine 25–50 mg IV/po

2. Continue to monitor patient carefully and frequently

3. Stop transfusion if symptoms worsen or additional symptoms develop

4. If uneventful, complete transfusion reaction investigation form

5. No need to send blood samples or blood bag

Temp increase by >1°C and >38°C	
1. Stop transfusion 2. Clerical check 3. Notify physician 4. Notify blood bank	
Clerical error or additional serious symptoms?	
No **Restart transfusion cautiously as ordered**	**Yes** **Do not restart transfusion**
1. Administer acetaminophen 325 mg 2. Continue to monitor patient carefully and frequently 3. Stop transfusion if symptoms worsen or additional symptoms develop 4. If uneventful, complete transfusion reaction investigation form 5. Send to blood bank with blood sample as per algorithm	1. Suspect hemolytic transfusion reaction or bacterial contamination 2. Initiate transfusion reaction investigation by completing form 3. Collect blood samples 4. Send blood bag to blood bank 5. Continue to monitor patient and report condition to physician

Table 5.
The protocol to follow in the case of emergence of fever during blood transfusion.

6. Infectious complications

6.1 Approximate risk per transfused unit of various infectious agents

The risk per transfused units for each infectious agent is as shown in **Table 6** [7].

Infectious agent	Approximate risk/transfused unit
Hepatitis B virus	1:750,000
Hepatitis C virus	1:1.1 million
HIV-1, HIV-2	1:2.7 million
Bacterial sepsis	1:75,000 (platelet transfusions)
Bacterial sepsis	1:250,000 to 1:10 million (red blood cell transfusions)

Table 6.
Infectious complications of transfusion.

6.2 Bacterial and parasitic transmissions by transfusion

In the United States, bacterial contamination of platelet products has been recognized as the most common cause of transfusion-associated morbidity and mortality owing to an infectious source. It exceeds hepatitis, HIV, and other viral sources put together. It was noted that the frequency of bacterial contamination is as high as 1 in 1000 to 1 in 2000 platelet units. It results in clinical sepsis after 1 in 4000 platelet transfusions before preventive measures were put in place. As an example, the introduction of bacterial screening has reduced the risk of septic transfusion reactions for apheresis platelets, and it has declined to approximately 1 in 75,000 with the risk of a fatal septic reaction declining to approximately 1 in 500,000 [7, 14, 15].

Efforts to detect the presence of bacteria in platelet units before dispensing to a patient include incubating an aliquot of the unit in a culture system and using a rapid strip immunoassay for bacterial antigens. Other less sensitive methods for detection using a surrogate marker for evidence of bacterial metabolism, such as a low pH, in an aliquot of the platelet suspension have been discontinued. While platelet products are typically contaminated by Gram-positive cocci, such as coagulase-negative Staphylococci, sepsis associated with transfusion of RBC units is most often due to Gram-negative organisms, particularly Yersinia enterocolitica.

Red blood cell contamination with Yersinia enterocolitica had resulted in bacteremia and septic shock which is often catastrophic. This Gram-negative organism can survive during refrigerated storage and lead to bacteremia or septic shock in the transfused recipient. Malarial transmission by transfusion is very common in Africa where malaria is known to be endemic but uncommon in Europe and America but cases are occasionally reported [7, 15].

6.3 Hepatitis

The estimated risk of post-transfusion hepatitis C is 1 per 1.1 million units transfused with current use of anti-hepatitis C virus antibody tests and nucleic acid testing.

Post transfusion hepatitis occasionally still develops despite the exclusive use of volunteer blood donors and screening of donor blood for hepatitis B and hepatitis C viruses. Transfusion-related hepatitis C virus infection is usually subclinical and anicteric in most cases but frequently becomes chronic and often results in clinically significant liver dysfunction [7, 15].

The risk of HBV transmission by transfusion decreased from 1:220,000 to approximately 1:750,000 after implementation of HBV DNA testing. Photochemical pathogen inactivation strategies appear both efficacious and relatively sparing in terms of qualitative platelet function, although decreases in quantitative platelet recovery have been observed in some studies [7, 15].

6.4 HIV and human T-cell lymphotropic viruses

The risk of acquiring HIV-1 or HIV-2 infection as a result of transfusion currently is estimated to be 1 in 1.5 million. Nucleic acid amplification testing for HIV has reduced the window of serologic conversion from 16 days to about 9 days. The use of heat-treated concentrates, solvent detergent-treated products, and recombinant factor concentrates has essentially eliminated HIV as a therapy-risk for hemophiliacs [7, 15].

6.5 Human T-cell lymphotropic virus 1 (HTLV-1)

This is a retrovirus associated with adult T-cell leukemia or lymphoma and tropical spastic paraparesis. Screening for HTLV-1 in blood donors is currently performed in the United States because asymptomatic blood donors can transmit this virus. Several cases of neuropathy had been reported in transfused recipients before the availability of testing.

HTLV-2, a related virus with antigenic cross-reactivity to HTLV-1, is endemic in certain Native American populations and also has been found in a high proportion of intravenous drug users. The risk of HTLV transmission by transfusion using current test methods is approximately 1 in 2.7 million [7, 15].

6.6 West Nile virus (WNV)

WNV became known to the US during the 2002 (WNV) epidemic in the United States wherein 23 individuals acquired WNV after blood transfusion. The characteristic clinical features manifested include fever, confusion, and encephalitis which developed within days to weeks of transfusion. As a result, blood centers implemented nucleic acid-based testing to screen all donations for WNV.

In a survey of 2.5 million donations in 2003, 601 donations (0.02%) were found to contain WNV. A subsequent follow-up study detected no cases of transfusion-transmitted WNV infection among recipients of tested blood; however, rare breakthrough transmissions have been reported [7, 15].

6.7 Parvovirus B19

Rare transmissions of parvovirus B19 by transfusion have been recognized. A recent study documented persistence of low levels of parvovirus B19 DNA in a high percentage of multi-transfused patients. The long-term clinical implications of this finding currently are unknown. Parvovirus (and other viruses without a lipid envelope such as hepatitis A virus) is not eliminated by solvent detergent treatment.

Acute parvovirus B19 infection can result in impaired erythropoiesis and can cause an aplastic crisis in patients with sickle cell disease and other hemolytic diseases. Infection with this virus can also result in significant fetal harm when a pregnant woman is infected during weeks 9–20 of pregnancy. There is no currently available blood donor screening assay for this virus [7, 15].

6.8 Cytomegalovirus (CMV)

CMV resides in leukocytes, and leukocytes inevitably contaminate RBC and platelet concentrate products. Hence, they are capable of transmitting CMV infection. Transfusion-transmitted CMV infection is an important issue in transfusion of cellular blood products to neonates, particularly low-birth-weight infants born to seronegative mothers, HSCT recipients, and other highly immunosuppressed patients [7, 15].

The risk of acquiring CMV from transfusions is particularly high when pre-transplantation serologic testing reveals that neither the HPSC donor nor the recipient has been previously exposed to CMV. In addition, transplantation recipients are at increased risk for transplantation-associated CMV reactivation when either the donor or the recipient is seropositive for CMV before transplantation. The latter consideration often affects the choice of HPSC donors. For these reasons, some institutions use blood products obtained exclusively from CMV-seronegative donors when providing blood products to neonatal recipients or recipients of HPSC transplantations.

However, as noted earlier, a landmark randomized comparison of leukoreduced versus CMV-seronegative blood components in CMV-seronegative HSCT recipients (with seronegative donors) found no significant difference in the incidence of CMV infection, and CMV disease as a composite outcome and most transplantation centers [7, 15].

In practice, prestorage leukoreduced blood components will be used for CMV prevention. Other institutions simply use leukoreduced blood products in all recipients, regardless of CMV status. The latter strategy has the additional advantage of reducing the risk of alloimmunization to HLA antigens and thus of developing refractoriness to platelet transfusions.

6.9 Parasites

Malaria: malarial transmission by transfusion is common in malarial endemic regions of Africa. In nonmalarial endemic areas, donors with a history of residence in a malaria-endemic area or travel associated with a risk of malarial exposure are deferred for up to 3 years, depending on the exposure.

Chagas disease: Trypanosoma cruzi parasites can survive several weeks of storage in blood, and contamination of blood products with this organism is already a significant problem in parts of South America. Therefore, the immigration of individuals from South America to the United States raises concerns that Chagas disease may emerge as a common transfusion-transmitted infection [7, 15].

An FDA-approved blood donor-screening test for antibodies to *T. cruzi* is available. Blood donors only need to be tested at their first donation.

Babesiosis: this has been identified in receiving platelets, refrigerated RBCs, and even frozen-thawed RBCs. Cases have been reported in New England and the upper Midwest. Various tests are being evaluated for donor screening in areas endemic for Babesia [7, 15].

7. Conclusions

This chapter serves as a synopsis to adverse blood reactions which are very common but apparently more often under-recognized and/or under-reported particularly in developing countries. This should sharpen the consciousness of all health practitioners involved in blood transfusion services towards taking measures at preventing transfusion reactions right from donor selection up to the infusion of blood into the recipients.

Conflict of interest

No conflict of interest.

Blood Transfusion Reactions
DOI: http://dx.doi.org/10.5772/intechopen.85347

Notes/Thanks/Other declarations

Chapter 12; Transfusion medicine: American Society of Hematology Self-Assessment Program served as a good template on which this chapter is built.

Author details

John Ayodele Olaniyi
College of Medicine, University College Hospital, University of Ibadan,
Ibadan, Nigeria

*Address all correspondence to: ayodeleolaniyi8@gmail.com

IntechOpen

References

[1] Tapko J, Mainuka P, Diarra-Nama AJ. Status of Blood Safety in the WHO African Region: Report of 2006 Survey. Brazaville, Republic of Congo: WHO Regional Office for Africa; 2006. Available from: http//wwwáfro.who.int/en/divisions-a-programmes/dsd/health-technologies-a-laboratories.html

[2] Suddock JT, Crookston K. Transfusion Reactions. StartPearls Publishing; 2018

[3] Land KJ, Townsend M, Goldman M, Whitaker BI, Perez GE, Wiersum-Osselton JC. International validation of harmonized definitions for complications of blood donations. Transfusion. 2018;**58**(11):2589-2595

[4] Webert K. Transfusion Reactions: Are Those Symptoms Normal? [PowerPoint slides]. 2015. Retrieved from http://www.transfusion.ca/

[5] Fung MK, editor. Non-infectious complications of blood transfusion. Chapter 27. In: AABB Technical Manual. 18th ed. Bethesda: AABB; 2014

[6] Popovsky M, editor. Transfusion Reactions. 3rd ed. Bethesda: AABB Press; 2007

[7] Savage W, Bakdash S. Transfusion medicine, Chapter 12. In: American Society of Haematology Self-Assessment Program Textbook. 6th ed. 2016. Available from: www.ash.sap.org

[8] Jasinski S, Glasser CL. Catastrophic delayed hemolytic transfusion reaction in a patient with sickle cell disease without alloantibodies: Case report and review of literature. Journal of Pediatric Hematology/Oncology. 2018. DOI 10.1097/MPH00000000001307. PMID: 30179992

[9] Fasano RM, Meyer EK, Branscomb J, White MS, Gibson RW, Eckman JR. Impact of red blood cell antigen matching on alloimmunization and transfusion complications in patients with sickle cell disease: A systematic review. Transfusion Medicine Reviews. 2018;**26**

[10] Siddon AJ, Kenney BC, Hendrickson JE, Tormey CA. Delayed haemolytic and serologic transfusion reactions: Pathophysiology, treatment and prevention. Current Opinion in Hematology. 2018;**25**(6):459-467

[11] Tariket S, Sut C, Hamzeh-Cognasse H, Laradi S, Garraud O, Cognasse F. Platelet and TRALI: From blood component to organism. Transfusion Clinique et Biologique. 2018;**25**(3):204-209

[12] Garraud O, Cognasse F, Laradi S, Hamzeh-Cognasse H, Peyrard T, Tissot JD, et al. How to mitigate the risk of inducing transfusion associated adverse reactions. Transfusion Clinique et Biologique. 2018;**25**(4):262-268

[13] Frazier SK, Higgins J, Bugajski A, Jones AR, Brown MR. Adverse reactions to transfusion of blood products and best practices for prevention. Critical Care Nursing Clinics of North America. 2017;**29**(3):271-290

[14] Erony SM, Marshall CE, Gehrie EA, Boyd JS, Ness PM, Tobian AAR, et al. The epidemiology of bacterial culture-positive and septic transfusion reactions at a large tertiary academic center: 2009 to 2016. Transfusion. 2018;**58**(8):1933-1939

[15] Block EM, Vermeuilen M, Murphy E. Blood transfusion safety in Africa: A literature of infectious diseases and organizational challenges. Transfusion Medicine Reviews. 2012;**26**(2):164-180. NIH Public Access authored Manuscript. DOI: 10.1016/j.tmrv.2011.07.006

Chapter 3

Hemolytic Disease of the Fetus and Newborn

Soumya Das

Abstract

Hemolytic disease of the fetus and newborn (HDFN) also called as "erythro-blastosis fetalis" is characterized by the increased rate of red blood cells (RBCs) destruction. Hemolysis should always be investigated even if the anemia is mild and apparently trivial. The principle clues which suggest hemolytic anemia includes: increased number of reticulocytes and/or circulating nucleated RBCs, unconjugated hyperbilirubinemia, a positive direct antiglobulin test and characteristic changes in red cells in the blood films. Based on etiology, hemolysis in newborn can be immune or non-immune mediated. The immune-mediated hemolysis due to blood group incompatibility between the mother and the fetus is the main cause of HDFN.

Keywords: hemolysis, blood groups

1. Introduction

Hemolytic disease of the fetus and newborn (HDFN) also called as "erythro-blastosis fetalis" is characterized by the increased rate of red blood cell (RBC) destruction. Hemolysis should always be investigated even if anemia is mild and apparently trivial. The principle clues which suggest hemolytic anemia include increased number of reticulocytes and/or circulating nucleated RBCs, unconjugated hyperbilirubinemia, a positive direct antiglobulin test, and characteristic changes in red cells in the blood films [1, 2]. Based on etiology, hemolysis in newborn can be immune or nonimmune mediated. The nonimmune causes include α-thalassemia, RBC membrane, or enzyme defects [1]. The immune-mediated hemolysis due to blood group incompatibility between the mother and the fetus is the main cause of HDFN. Immune-mediated hemolysis of fetal red cells, due to blood group incompatibility, occurs when there is transplacental passage of maternal antibody active against paternal red cell antigen of the infant [2–4]. Both naturally occurring and immune antibodies are implicated leading to a spectrum of clinical sequela, ranging from anemia and hyperbilirubinemia to fetal hydrops, kernicterus, and death [3, 4]. Although more than 60 different RBC antigens are capable of eliciting an antibody response, significant morbidity is associated primarily with D antigen of Rh group [2]. The prevalence of red cell antibodies other than anti-D with the potency to induce HDFN is about 1 in 500 pregnancies [5–7].

2. History

The royal family of England was not spared from the features of HDFN. Henry VIII's first wife, *Katherine of Aragon*, conceived six times, among which five died in the perinatal period due to features presumed to be of HDFN [8]. The well-documented description of HDFN was made in 1609 by the midwife in the French literature. The case was a twin gestation in which the first fetus was stillborn and the second twin developed jaundice and succumbed soon after birth [9]. In 1940, Rh blood group system was described by Landsteiner and Wiener, and in 1941 Levine et al. determined that D antigen in Rh system is the agent for HDFN [10, 11]. The main cause of sensitization though was stated by Levine in 1940 but was described in detail by Keenan and Pearse in 1963 [12]. In 1961 Liley, for the first time, described intrauterine transfusion into the abdominal cavity of the fetus as a preventive measure for the disease [13]. Exchange transfusion, introduced by Wallerstein, and induced premature delivery are other treatment options employed for the management of HDFN [14, 15]. Until 1960, HDFN due to rhesus blood group system was considered the major contributor to the perinatal mortality rates. In 1961, Finn et al. defined the administration of anti-D Ig in the prevention of Rh sensitization and later in 1967 along with two German scientists Schneider and Preisler proved that anti-D is not useful in already sensitized mothers [16, 17]. This was a major breakthrough in prevention of sensitization with administration of 400 μg of human anti-D globulin within 72 h after delivery. Since 1971, the WHO recommends empirical use of anti-D Ig following any sensitizing event including after delivery of Rh-positive newborn and for abortions.

3. Blood group antigens and antibodies

An antigen is any substance which, when introduced into the body of an immunocompetent individual, stimulates the immune system by production of an antibody by interacting with the immunoglobulin receptor of B cell. Each red cell membrane is a bi-phospholipid layer containing millions of antigen on its surface [18]. The blood group antigens are either protein or carbohydrate structures present on the red cell membrane. An individual's blood group is determined by the antigen expressed on the surface of red cell membrane. The carbohydrate antigens are expressed as it is, while the protein antigens stretch in the bi-phospholipid layer by transmembrane proteins [19].

Antibodies are recognition proteins found in the serum and other body fluids of vertebrates that react specifically with the antigens that induce their formation. Antibodies belong to a family of globular proteins called immunoglobulins. The terms antibody and immunoglobulins are used synonymously. They are produced by the lymphocyte-plasma cell system. Antibodies bind antigen, fix complement, facilitate phagocytosis, and neutralize toxic substances in the circulation [18]. IgG, IgM, and IgA are the most significant from the point of view of transfusion medicine. Most clinically significant antibodies are IgG type, reacting at body temperature (37°C) with the antigens, and cause significant in transfusion reactions as they are a class of antibodies produced in response to nonself-antigens on the blood products. IgM antibodies are mostly naturally occurring antibodies [19].

4. Alloimmunization during pregnancy

Alloimmunization can be caused due to pregnancy, blood transfusion, or tissue/organ transplantation or grafting, due to genetic difference between the individuals [20]. On exposure to a foreign red cell antigen, the immune system is activated which is mediated by lymphocytes. The first step involved is recognition of the antigen by T cell. The recipient's helper T cell interacts with the MHC class II

Antepartum	Intrapartum	Postpartum
Early pregnancy	Caesarean section	Blood transfusion
Abortion (spontaneous or induced)	Manual removal of placenta	
Ectopic pregnancy		
Late pregnancy		
Placetal abruption		
Abodominal trauma		
Obstetric procedures		
Amniocentesis		
Chorionic villus sampling		
External cephalic version		
Fetal blood sampling		

Table 1.
Sensitizing events for feto-maternal haemorrhage [24].

molecule expressed on the donor red cells. Following the initial interaction, T cells trigger a second signal for the B lymphocytes, in order to stimulate humoral immune response [20, 21]. Initially, IgM class of antibody is produced in primary response to an antigen and is formed as early as 4 weeks to 3 months period. However, there is a switch of IgM to IgG class during the secondary response [20]. The secondary response is more rapid, potent, and specific than the primary.

Placenta is a natural barrier present between mother and fetus. Only IgG antibodies can cross the placenta. The transfer is mediated by the neonatal Fc receptors (FcRn) [6]. The immunoglobulin is bound and transported by FcRn of syncytiotrophoblast which also protects IgG molecule from normal serum protein catabolism. In the first trimester, there is relatively less transfer; however, it subsequently increases exponentially in the second and third trimester. Mean concentration in the fetus at the 24th week of pregnancy is 1.8 g/dL. The IgG antibody levels are higher in the fetus than in the mother toward the term [22]. Of the four subclasses of IgG antibody, IgG3 and IgG1 are more efficient in RBC hemolysis than IgG2 and IgG4, though all the four classes are efficiently transferred across the placenta [23].

4.1 Sensitizing events

Transplacental feto-maternal hemorrhage occurs in over 75% of pregnancies. The average volume of fetal blood in the maternal circulation following delivery is less than 1 mL in 96% of pregnancies [24]. As the pregnancy progresses, the possibility of feto-maternal hemorrhage increases, 3% in first trimester, 12% in the second, 45% in the third, and 64% at the time of delivery as shown by Bowman [22]. It has been reported that as little as 0.1 mL of antigen-positive blood is sufficient to cause sensitization in an antigen-negative mother [23]. Feto-maternal hemorrhage can occur due to various antenatal and postnatal events in **Table 1**.

5. Pathophysiology for HDFN

HDFN is the destruction of fetal and newborn red cells by maternal alloantibodies specific for the inherited paternal red cell alloantigens. While IgM is usually detected in the maternal circulation during primary response, IgG is found during secondary response, which appears about 5–15 weeks after feto-maternal hemorrhage. Because exposure to fetal red cells and resulting maternal alloimmunization typically occurs late during pregnancy and at delivery, and IgM does not cross the placenta, the fetus and newborn of the first pregnancy are rarely affected. Re-exposure to red cell antigen during subsequent pregnancies produces IgG in sufficient concentration [4].

The sensitized fetal red cells by maternal IgG antibody are unable to continue in the circulation, and these red cells are destroyed by the fetal spleen resulting in anemia. Compensatory erythropoiesis is induced by fetal anemia initially [25]. The exception to this rule is antibodies Kell blood group system and MNS system which cause destruction of erythroid progenitor cells, causing early anemia without erythroblastosis [26, 27]. Hyperdynamic circulation tries to compensate anemia in the fetus, which subsequently leads to cardiomegaly, and finally fetal hydrops develops [25]. Due to hemolysis of the fetal cell, there is rise in the bilirubin level in the fetus. In utero, the bilirubin is excreted by the mother, when it is transported across the placenta, so the severity of hyperbilirubinemia is not observed. After delivery, the hemolysis continues, but the comparatively immature liver of the neonate is unable to sufficiently conjugate the excess of bilirubin. This subsequently leads to severe hyperbilirubinemia and, when left untreated, could result in "kernicterus" [4, 25, 28].

6. Clinical relevance of different red cell alloantibody specificities

The risk of developing severe HDFN depends on several factors, including Ig class, specificity of the red cell alloantibodies, and level of expression of the involved blood group antigen on the fetal red cells and other tissues as shown in **Table 2** [25].

6.1 Rh blood group system

Rh system is more complex than the single antigen system. Five principal Rh antigens D, C, c, E, and e are responsible for the majority of clinically significant antibodies, but over 50 different Rh antigens have been described [29].

Antibody specificities	Risk to develop HDFN in antigen-positive children and clinical course of disease
ABO	Low risk for disease, in general mild, incidentally severe
Rh D c E Other Rh antigens	High risk for disease, often (very) severe, otherwise mild High risk for disease, (very) severe or mild Medium risk for disease, sometimes severe, but mostly mild Medium risk for disease, incidentally severe, but mostly mild
Kell K Other Kell antigens	High risk for disease, (very) severe or mild Medium risk mild to severe disease
Duffy Fya/Fyb	Medium risk for disease, mostly mild
Kidd Jka/Jkb	Low risk for disease, only mild
MNS M, N, S, s Other antigens	Low risk for disease, mostly mild disease, very rarely severe Low risk for disease, mostly mild disease, very rarely severe
I, Le, P1, Lu, Yt	No risk, because of very low expression of these antigens by fetal cells
Other antigen systems	Very low risk, very rarely severe disease can develop

Table 2.
Red cell antibody specificities in reference to induce HDFN [25].

D is by far the most immunogenic of all the Rh antigens. Hence, it is common in clinical practice to equate D with Rh and to use the terms Rh-positive and Rh-negative to describe "D-positive" and "D-negative" [30].

Rh antibodies implicated in HDFN are:

- Severe HDFN—anti-D and anti-c [31, 32]

- Mild disease—anti-C, anti-E, and anti-e [33–37]

6.1.1 D antigen and antibodies

The D antigen carried by the RhD proteins is the most immunogenic and most important blood group antigen leading to HDFN. There is no antithetical antigen to D [4]. The first blood group antigen to be associated with HDFN was described by Levine et al. in 1945 [9]. About 15% of Western world and 8% of blacks are D-negative [38, 39]. If a unit of D-positive blood is transfused to a D-negative recipient, the recipient will form anti-D in around 90% of cases, and subsequently D-positive red cells cannot be given safely to these patients [29].

Sensitization to D antigen can occur in reaction to less than 0.1 mL of fetal blood, resulting in formation of anti-D in the maternal circulation [22]. Before 1945, more than 50% of all fetus with HDFN died of kernicterus or hydrops fetalis, and anti-D was the most common associated [9, 40]. With improvement of treatment, in industrialized countries the mortality reduced to 2–3%. But anti-D is still among the most frequently detected antibodies in sensitized pregnancies.

Very early, it was understood that, if the D-negative mother was carrying an ABO-compatible D-positive fetus, her risk of Rh immunization was 16%. If the D-positive fetus was ABO-incompatible, the risk was only 2%. So, the overall risk of Rh immunization is 13.2% [9].

Not only in Rh-negative pregnancies does anti-D causes HDFN, but also case reports have been reported for HDFN due to anti-D in Rh-positive pregnancies [41–43]. These are mostly due to the Rh variants: weak D, Du, and partial D described by molecular analysis [30].

6.1.1.1 Blocked D phenomenon

The blocking of D antigen sites by IgG anti-D in severe cases of HDFN is a rare phenomenon explained by Wiener in 1944 [44]. Only a handful of case reports have been described in the literature [45–48]. The coating of maternal anti-D IgG on the D-positive red blood cells (RBCs) of the newborn gives false-negative D typing, when IgM typing reagent anti-D is used. This phenomenon is not limited to anti-D, but is seen with other blood groups [49]. BCSH describes guideline for resolving such cases [50].

6.1.1.2 Rh immunoglobulin prophylaxis

Rh immunoglobulin (RhIG) prophylaxis for D-negative pregnant women is now the international cornerstone for prevention of maternal alloimmunization to the D antigen and subsequent HDFN [50, 51].

During the mid-1960s, experiments were carried out in various parts of the world for preventing HDFN due to anti-D. Clinical trials showed that, when unimmunized mothers who have delivered D-positive infants, were given RhIG prevented the development of anti-D in the mother. RhIG is obtained from the human plasma. RhIG has to be given within 72 h after delivery of a D-positive infant. Since 1968, RhIG is licensed for prevention of HDFN [9, 21, 22].

The effectiveness of RhIG in order to prevent isoimmunization is determined by adequate dosage and should be administered before initiation of Rh isoimmunization [50].

There are various mechanisms describing the role of RhIG in preventing HDFN. Though antigenic epitopes are not fully masked by anti-D, they are still available for immune system recognition. But anti-D is be able to destroy RBCs without triggering the adaptive immune response, by inhibition of FcgammaRIIB signaling in B cells which is called as antibody-mediated immune suppression (AMIS) [21, 52, 53]. The T-cell response and memory may still be intact.

Various studies were carried out in the 1970s after systemic implementation of systemic anti-D prophylaxis, which showed reduction in HDFN from 16 to 0.3% [54].

The standard guidelines recommend to administer RhIG as soon after delivery as the infant is determined to be D-positive or latest within 72 hours after delivery or after any antenatal procedure, where the risk of feto-maternal hemorrhage is high as shown in **Table 3** [50]. It has been shown experimentally that at least partial protection is afforded by giving RhIG up to 13 days after exposure to D-positive RBCs. Rh prophylaxis therefore is recommended up to 28 days after delivery, with the understanding, however, that the longer the prophylaxis after delivery is delayed, the less likely it is to be effective [28, 55].

In 2014, Cohen et al. described a case report on severe HDFN caused due to passive transfer of anti-D from maternal RhIG [56].

6.1.2 Other Rh system antibodies other than anti-D

With widespread use of RhD immunoglobulin, the focus has shifted to the non-RhD antibodies causing isoimmunization. Other Rh antigens include C, c, E, and e antigens. DCe is the most common haplotype in Caucasians (42%), Native Americans (44%), and Asians (70%) [57].

6.1.3 Anti-c

Anti-c is usually described as the next most common cause of severe HDFN after anti-D. Various case reports have been reported, stating that anti-c isoimmunization can cause HDFN from mild to severe degree [31, 32, 58, 59]. A titer of more than 1:32 is associated with hydrops fetalis as described by David et al. [58]. BCSH guidelines state that women with anti-c should be retested following the same protocol as for anti-D [50]. Quantification of the antibodies is expressed in terms of IU/mL. Mothers with antibody concentration of less than 7.5 IU/mL are advised to continue the pregnancy, while 7.5–20 IU/mL are at a risk of moderate HDFN and more than 20 IU/mL, severe HDFN. It should be kept in mind that anti-c causes delayed anemia in neonate [50].

6.1.4 Anti-D + anti-C or anti-G

D-positive or C-positive RBCs have G antigen which was first described by Allen and Tippett in 1958 [60]. The G antigen is co-distributed either with C or D antigen which causes anti-G to appear serologically as anti-C plus anti-D [60]. During pregnancy, it is apparently important to distinguish between anti-D, anti-G, and anti-D + C. As the pregnancies without anti-D are candidates for the administration

Recommendations	Strength of recommendation	Quality of evidence
Postpartum prophylaxis	A	I
• Anti-D 120–300 μg within 72 h of delivery	B	II
• Anti-D up to 28 days after delivery	C	Insufficient
• Routine FMH testing after delivery		
Antepartum prophylaxis	A	I
• Anti-D 300 μg at 28 weeks	C	III
• Repeat antibody screening at 28 weeks	C	III
• Routine paternal testing	D	III
• Anti-D for "weak D" (e.g., Du)	D	III
• Repeat anti-D at 40 weeks		
Early pregnancy loss and termination	B	II-3
• Anti-D 120–300 μg after spontaneous/induced	B	III
abortion	B	III
• Antibody screening prior to anti-D after abortion	B	III
• Ectopic pregnancy: 120–300 μg Rh immune globulin		
• Molar pregnancy: 120–300 μg Rh immune globulin		
Invasive fetal procedures	B	II-3
• Amniocentesis: 300 μg Rh immune globulin	B	II
• CVS: 120–300 μg Rh immune globulin	B	II-3
• Cordocentesis: 300 μg Rh immune globulin		
APH, abdominal trauma, ECV, FMH	B	III
• Quantitative FMH testing	B	III
• Anti-D 120–300 μg following placental trauma		
Consent	C	III
• Informed consent prior to administration of anti-D		

Table 3.
Anti-D prophylaxis and quality of evidence available [50, 54, 55].

of RhIG. The administration of RhIG can be avoided if anti-D has already developed. D-negative mothers with anti-G are potential candidates to receive RhIG in order to prevent formation of anti-D. It also avoids the associated social or medicolegal complications [61]. The clinical significance of anti-G alone in causing mild to severe HDFN still remains controversial [62]. The isolation of anti-G by double adsorption and elution is a tedious and relatively complex procedure [63]. The technique to distinguish anti-D + C from anti-G is recently described by Fatima et al. [64].

6.1.5 Anti-C, anti-E, anti-e, and others

Anti-RhC, anti-RhE, and anti-Rhe antibodies are of Rhesus family and usually occur in low titer in conjunction with anti-RhD antibody. Their presence can be additive to the hemolytic effect of the anti-RhD on the fetus [65, 66]. Various reports have been published on pregnancies alloimmunized only to RhE [36, 37].

Hardy and Napier in their review of red blood cell antibodies among Rh-positive women in South and Mid Wales over a 30-year period (1948–1978) described two infants with hemolytic disease caused by anti-C [67].

Anti-e is usually a very rare cause of HDN; the disease is usually mild [68].

In addition to the above antibodies, there are many other antibodies belonging to Rh family which are associated with HDFN [35, 69, 70].

6.2 Kell blood group system

A mnemonic goes "Duffy dies, Kell kills, and Lewy lives" [71]. Kell blood group system is clinically significant in terms of transfusion medicine and perinatology. It relates to the polymorphic nature of the Kell protein. It is also associated with the Kx and Gerbich blood group systems. K is formed in fetuses of 10–11 weeks and k at 6–7 weeks of gestation [72, 73].

Alloimmunization to Kell blood group antigens is due to previous blood transfusion or feto-maternal hemorrhage induced during pregnancy [73]. Kell alloimmunization is the second major cause for fetal hemolytic anemia, with a reported and still increasing incidence in a large US series of 3.2 in 1000 and affecting 1 in 10,000 neonates [74].

6.2.1 Anti-K

Anti-K antibodies differ from the other blood group system antibodies that cause HDFN in suppressing fetal non-hemoglobinized erythropoiesis, causing severe anemia and often death of the fetus. The high bilirubin level is not a characteristic feature as the precursor cells are destroyed. Amniocentesis therefore does not give an indication of the severity of the disease. Successful management of RBC-alloimmunized pregnancies depends on early detection of fetal anemia and timely intervention by intrauterine blood transfusions [75–77].

Perinatal survival in severe Kell alloimmunization was only 58% as recorded after implementation of routine screening nationwide in the Netherlands from 1988 to 2005 [75].

In some countries it is usually practiced to give K-negative red cells for girls and women of childbearing age group [78].

6.3 Detection of feto-maternal hemorrhage (FMH)

6.3.1 KB test

As mentioned earlier, feto-maternal hemorrhage increases as the pregnancy progresses: 3% in the first trimester, 12% in the second, 45% in the third, and 64% at the time of delivery [22]. These fetal cells which have crossed the placenta can be detected by acid elution method of differential staining described by Kleinhauer and Betke in 1960 [79].

6.3.2 α-Fetoprotein (α-FP)

α-FP is an analogue of albumin [6]. Seppala and Ruoslahti in 1972 and Caballero et al. in 1977 used α-FP as an index of transplacental hemorrhage (TPH) [80, 81].

6.3.3 Others

Apart from quantification, the serological methods for detecting transplacental hemorrhage are also available. This includes rosetting test and flow cytometry.

Rosetting test is not sensitive, as it needs at least 15 mL or more of fetal cells to be present in the maternal circulation to give a positive result [19].

Flow cytometry is the most sensitive test technique in detecting the amount of TPH [19, 82].

The other surrogate markers of FMH include enzyme-linked antiglobulin test (ELAT), placental alkaline phosphatase (PLAP), polymerase chain reaction (PCR), and fluorescence in situ hybridization (FISH).

6.4 Antibody screening

It had been a common practice to screen the sera of all Rh(D)-negative pregnant women for Rh antibodies. Later, when it was found that Rh(D)-positive women could also have babies with HDFN due to Rh antibodies (other than anti-D) and non-Rh antibodies, it was suggested that sera from all pregnant women should be screened for antibodies [6, 25, 83].

6.4.1 Screening methods

The indirect antiglobulin test (IAT) using reagent red cells suspended in low ionic strength saline (LISS) is the most suitable method for detection of clinically significant red cell antibodies [84]. Column agglutination methods, liquid-phase tube tests, and solid-phase methods have also been found to be suitable [50].

6.4.2 Guidelines for antenatal antibody screening

Various countries have developed guidelines for screening of antenatal cases. Scientific Section Coordinating Committee of the American Association of Blood Banks (AABB) has issued guidelines (not AABB standards) for serological testing of pregnant women [85]. **Table 4** shows the recommendations for prenatal testing.

The BCSH Task Force has also laid guidelines in 2007 for blood grouping and antibody testing in pregnancy as follows [50]:

Testing and condition	Timing
ABO	Initial visit
First pregnancy	Initial visit
Subsequent pregnancies	For pretransfusion testing
Other	
Rh (test for weak D optional)	Initial visit and at 26–28 weeks' gestation
First pregnancy	Initial visit
Subsequent pregnancies	For pretransfusion testing
Other	
Unexpected antibodies	Initial visit
All pregnancies	Before Rh Ig therapy (optional)
D− pregnancies	Third trimester if transfused or history of unexpected
D+ pregnancies	antibodies
Other	For pretransfusion testing
Antibody identification	Upon initial detection
Unexpected antibodies present	At time of titration
Confirmatory testing	
Antibody titration	Upon initial detection
Rh antibodies	Repeat at 18–20 weeks' gestation
Other potentially significant	Repeat at 2- to 4-week intervals if below critical titer [16–32]
antibodies	As above, with discussion with obstetrician

Table 4.
AABB recommendations for prenatal testing [85].

- "*All pregnant women* should have samples taken early in pregnancy, ideally at 10–16 weeks gestation, for ABO and D typing and for screening for the presence of red cell alloantibodies."

- "All pregnant women, *whether D-positive or -negative* should have a further blood sample taken at 28 weeks gestation for rechecking the ABO and D group and further screening for red cell alloantibodies."

- "No further routine blood grouping or antibody screening is necessary *after 28 weeks of gestation.*"

Australian and New Zealand guidelines have been adapted from AABB recommendations for pregnant women [85, 86]. However, repeat testing of RhD-negative women only at 28 weeks, prior to administering RhIG, is becoming the accepted protocol in most Australian centers, eliminating the norm of antibody screening at 34–36 weeks. In New Zealand, in the absence of routine antenatal prophylaxis, the normal practice is to test RhD-negative women at 28 and 36 weeks of gestation [86].

The latest guidelines for alloimmunized pregnancy framed and followed in Japan since 2014 are as follows [87]:

- "Identify the antibody when a screening test, such as the indirect Coombs test, suggests the presence of an atypical antibody against red blood cells."

- "Assess the titer of the antibody if the antibody belongs to IgG class that may cause hemolysis in the fetus."

- "Monitor the fetal well-being, paying special attention to anemia and hydrops, in women with an elevated titer of an IgG antibody that may cause hemolysis in the fetus."

- "Be prepared to administer un-crossmatched packed red blood cells compatible with an ABO blood type if the pregnant woman develops unexpected massive bleeding."

6.5 Methods of red cell antibody detection and identification

Antibody detection plays a critical role in detection and monitoring of antenatal cases who are at risk of delivering neonates with HFDN [88].

Most of the clinically significant antibodies are IgG in nature, which are non-agglutinating or incomplete antibodies, so they can only sensitize red cells but cannot produce agglutination. Coombs et al. in 1945 described "antiglobulin test" for detection of these non-agglutinating antibodies [89].

The presence of red cell antibodies in patient's serum or plasma and an in vitro reaction between red cell detection are demonstrated by indirect antiglobulin test [89]. Indirect antiglobulin test is considered to be the most effective and reliable method for detection of clinically significant antibodies [84]. Several studies have shown that the column agglutination test is better than tube and solid-phase tests.

The gel technique has shown sensitivity as compared with conventional test tube (CTT) methods (93.5–100% for CAT vs. 50% for CTT) [90–93]. The sensitivity of SPRCA has been found to be superior to CTT and comparable with that of CAT [94].

6.6 Quantification of antibody in the serum

Titration is a semiquantitative method to estimate the strength and concentration of antibodies present in a serum sample [95]. Titers give only rough estimates of the amount of antibody bound to the target RBCs and do not measure the amount of antibody remaining free in solution at the endpoint of agglutination [96]:

- The critical titer for anti-D (the level below which HDFN and hydrops fetalis are considered unlikely is usually 16 or 32 in antihuman globulin (AHG) phase). These titer criteria apply to anti-D, to other Rh antibodies, and generally to other clinically significant antibodies, with anti-K as possible exception.

- A critical titer of 8 is considered for anti-K.

- As long as the titer is 8 or lower (except anti-K), the pregnancy can be followed up every 4–6 weeks until delivery.

- A difference of two dilutions or a score of 10 is considered a significant change [4].

- A score may also be assigned, based on the strength of reactivity.

- Each reaction is given a value, and score is determined by adding up individual values.

- Most hospitals have set up their critical antibody titer, at which amniocentesis is recommended.

There are various methods of performing the titration, conventional tube test (CTT), or by gel microcolumn assay (GMA) [95, 97]. A study by Thakur et al. showed that gel technique is more sensitive for antibody detection. It does not show a linear correlation with tube titers in predicting the outcome in RhD-sensitized women, while Rachel et al. suggested that GMA gives comparable results to the CTT in titrating alloantibodies to Rh and Kell antigens [95, 97].

6.7 Amniotic fluid analysis

Amniocentesis is helpful in determining the overall condition of the fetus and is mostly indicated when the clinically significant maternal antibody titer is 1:32 or greater in the fourth or fifth month of pregnancy [4, 19, 98]. If there is a history of a previous pregnancy complicated by HDN, amniocentesis is indicated regardless of the present maternal serum antibody titer.

In 1961, Liley developed a chart depicting change in amniotic fluid bilirubin levels (delta OD450) with period of gestation, with three zones delineating the severity of rhesus disease [99]. The chart is useful only after the 27th week of gestation. Currently, cordocentesis is the only reliable means of assessing the fetal condition accurately prior to 27 weeks. In 1993, Queenan proposed a chart showing delta OD450 from 14 to 40 weeks, with four zones to guide management [100].

6.8 Other methods for assessing the severity of HDFN

6.8.1 Ultrasound

Some of the pathophysiological changes in the fetus due to anemia could be shown using ultrasound [6]. Real-time sonography accurately predicted the clinical course in 86% of the cases, with no false-positive predictions [101].

With recent advances, Doppler ultrasonography, which measures fetal hemodynamics, has been used, and it gives better results in predicting fetal anemia as early as the 18th week. The Doppler assessment of peak systolic velocity in the middle cerebral artery (MCA-PSV) is done [102]. It is hypothesized that faster rate of blood flow indicates a more severely anemic fetus, with severe anemia being an indicator of fetal hydrops.

6.8.2 Fetoscopy, percutaneous umbilical blood sampling (cordocentesis), and chorionic villus biopsy

Fetoscopy is a technique in which the second-trimester fetus can be visualized directly and fetal blood (or other tissues) can be sampled through an endoscope introduced transabdominally into the amniotic cavity. The technique is only reliably successful at 16 weeks of gestation and later. Fetoscopy carries a mortality rate of 5% as compared to a 1–2% mortality rate after midtrimester amniocentesis. The fetal blood can be tested for blood type, DAT, hemoglobin, and hematocrit [96]. MacKenzie and coworkers suggested that the technique would be of benefit in cases where the father of the baby is known to be heterozygous for the offending blood group antigen in the following situations:

1. Patients with a history of previous babies having severe HDFN.

2. Patients with high-titer anti-D (e.g., in excess of 20 IU/mL) during the first 20 weeks of pregnancy.

6.8.3 Prenatal determination of fetal blood groups

The father's probable genotype is predicted. If the father is thought to be homozygous, the baby is assumed to possess the putative antigen. If the father is heterozygous, there is a 50% chance that the baby is antigen-positive [6, 96]. Antenatal genotyping of the fetus is now in widespread use as an aid to the clinical management in cases where there is a possibility of occurancy of hemolytic disease of the newborn [121]. Molecular genotyping is a major clinical application which has led to the determination basis of blood group antigens expressed, most of which have been defined at the level of the gene. All assays used are dependent on the polymerase chain reaction amplification of fetal DNA derived from.

6.8.4 In vitro predictive tests utilizing functional cellular assays

They are based on the in vivo mechanisms of RBC immune destruction. The interactions with the monocytes are measured by recording RBC adherence/phagocytosis by a monocyte monolayer assay (MMA), antibody-dependent cellular cytotoxicity (ADCC) using 51Cr-labeled RBCs, or a chemiluminescence test (CL) using luminol. These tests are not very accurate in predicting the severity of HDFN [6, 96].

6.9 Antenatal treatment of hemolytic disease

6.9.1 Plasma exchange in mother

A known therapeutic approach for red cell alloimmunization is plasmapheresis in the mother in order to reduce maternal antibody titer [103]. In the current era, plasma exchange treatment appears to be useful in cases of HDFN developed early in pregnancy (before 20 weeks). The American Society for Apheresis in 2013 proposed that plasmapheresis should be considered early in pregnancy (from the 7th to the 20th week) and continued until IUT can be safely administered (approx. 20 weeks of gestation) [104].

6.9.2 Absorption of alloantibodies onto red cells

Plasma containing the antibodies is drawn from the patient, the antibodies are absorbed using appropriate cells, and then plasma is returned to the patient [19]. During the 1980s, this procedure was attempted by Robinson and Yoshida et al. for an Rh-immunized woman [105, 106].

6.9.3 Intravenous immunoglobulin given to the mother

The use of intravenous immunoglobulin (IVIG) to the mother is one of the alternative strategies developed in past 20 years for the management of severely alloimmunized pregnancies [107]. The mechanism by which IVIG might act is saturation of FcRn, thereby inhibiting placental transfer of anti-D to the fetus as shown by Morgan et al. in 1991 [108]. A single course of 2 g/kg over 5 days or repeated weekly injections of 1 g/kg have been tried in conjunction with plasma exchange or with intravascular transfusion of the fetus [109]. There is no other description of the dosing during the antenatal period.

6.9.4 IVIG given to the fetus

IVIG given to the fetus did not show any beneficial effect [19].

6.9.5 Intrauterine transfusion

In 1970, Pontuch stated five strategies as a preventive measure for HDFN, which are valid to this day [110]:

1. "Prevention of leakage of fetal erythrocytes into maternal circulation and antibodies in the opposite direction"

2. "Blockage of antibody production in the maternal circulation"

3. "Prevention of sensitization of maternal erythrocytes with fetal erythrocytes"

4. "Prevention of Rh sensitization by anti-D administration"

5. "Intrauterine transfusion in pregnancy"

One of the oldest methods, introduced by *Sir William Liley*, is intraperitoneal fetal blood transfusion into the abdominal cavity of the fetus under X-ray guidance [111]. The donor cells were absorbed into the fetal circulation via the subdiaphragmatic lymphatics and thoracic duct, which, in conjunction with the use of amniotic fluid analysis for bilirubin levels, markedly improved the management of Rh-sensitized pregnancies.

From the time of its initiation, IUT has come a long way. Initially, it was intraperitoneal, but in 1981, Rodeck et al. described intravascular transfusion by using the umbilical cord and fetoscope [112].

The formula for calculation of blood volume for IUT is shown below [113]:

$$V = \frac{(\text{Desired PCV–Fetal PCV}) \times \text{Fetoplacental BV}}{(\text{Donor PCV–Desired PCV})}.$$

Red cell prerequisites for IUT as described by BCSH guidelines are as follows [113]:

- "Group O (low titre haemolysin) or ABO identical with the fetus (if known) and RhD negative"

- "IAT-cross-match compatible with maternal serum and negative for the relevant antigens determined by maternal antibody status"

- "Less than 5 days old and in citrate phosphate dextrose (CPD) anticoagulant"

- "CMV seronegative and irradiated"

- "Should have a haematocrit (packed cell volume, PCV) of up to but not more than 0.75"

- "Not be transfused straight from 4°C storage"

- "The rate of transfusion should be 5–10 mL/min"

The target of a single IUT is to reach Hct 48–55% in non-hydropic fetuses [103].

6.9.6 Induction of GvHD

Immunomodulatory effect due to transfusion to the fetus by IUT due to the HLA group of the donor causes GvHD [19].

6.9.7 Premature delivery

Premature induction of labor may be considered, as after the birth of the infant, placental transfer of antibody ceases [6, 28].

6.10 Postnatal intervention for hemolytic disease

6.10.1 Exchange transfusion

The main purposes of exchange transfusion in HDFN are as follows [28, 114]:

1. With sedimented red cells, it can raise the hematocrit without increasing the blood volume of a severely affected erythroblastotic newborn infant in the first minutes of life.

2. It can remove antibody-coated cells from the circulation of newborn before they hemolyze and produce bilirubin.

3. It can remove bilirubin in the circulating plasma and some from extravascular areas, so that its concentration can be kept below levels which are generally considered to be toxic to tissues—particularly central nervous system tissues.

The method was introduced by Diamond (1947). Blood was withdrawn and injected, intermittently, through a plastic catheter passed up the umbilical vein [110].

For HDFN double-volume exchange is mostly preferred, where approximately 85% of the blood volume is replaced and will cause an approximate reduction of 50% in pre-exchange bilirubin level [114–116]. The American Academy of Pediatrics (AAP) has published guidelines, recommending not to initiate early ET, such as within the first 12 h of birth. The bilirubin threshold for the start of ET depends on the gestational age at which the baby is born [117].

Components used in exchange transfusion.

Red cells for exchange transfusion should meet the following BCSH criteria [113, 118]:

- "Group O or ABO compatible with maternal and neonatal plasma, RhD negative (or RhD identical with neonate)"

- "Negative for any red cell antigens to which the mother has antibodies"

- "IAT-cross-match compatible with maternal plasma"

- "5 days old or less (to ensure optimal red cell function and low supernatant potassium levels)"

- "Collected into CPD anticoagulant and CMV seronegative"

- "Irradiated and transfused within 24 h of irradiation. Irradiation is essential if the infant has had a previous IUT and is recommended for all ETs"

- "Hematocrit of 0.50–0.60"

- "Not to be transfused straight from 4°C storage. Care should be taken to avoid over-heating of the component"

Fresh frozen plasma (FFP)—The RBCs are suspended in AB plasma in order to provide plasma proteins, coagulation factors, and albumin [113]. Reconstituted whole blood is prepared by adding appropriate amount of FFP into the RBC unit which is preservative-free. The hematocrit of the unit should be 40–45% [119]. Volume of blood for exchange is calculated using an estimate of the neonate's circulating blood volume [113]:

- Term infants: 80–160 mL/kg

- Preterm infants: 100–200 mL/kg

$$\boxed{\text{Volume to be exchange} = 2 \times \text{circulating blood volume}}$$

The volume to be given is calculated below [119]:

Total volume (in mL) = infant's weight in kg $\times$ 85* mL/kg $\times$ 2
Absolute volume of RBCs required (in mL) = total volume $\times$ 0.45 (desired hematocrit)
Actual volume of RBCs required (in mL) = $\dfrac{\text{Absolute volume}}{\text{Hematocrit of unit after any manipulation}}$
Necessary volume of FFP = total volume required − actual volume of RBCs required
$*$(85–100 mL/kg, depending on estimated blood volume)

6.10.2 Phototherapy

Phototherapy has been proven to be effective in treatment of hyperbilirubinemia by denaturing the bilirubin at appropriate wavelength [28]. AAP and NICE have laid down guidelines for initiation of treatment, considering gestational age, birth weight, and cause of hyperbilirubinemia [117, 120].

6.10.3 Intravenous immunoglobulin

IVIG blocks the Fc receptor sites on the cells of the reticuloendothelial system, thus preventing the hemolysis of sensitized cells. It is mostly used for ABO HDFN and is not very effective in anti-D-mediated HDFN [25, 28].

Author details

Soumya Das
Department of Transfusion Medicine, Jawaharlal Institute of Postgraduate Medical Education and Research (JIPMER), Pondicherry, India

*Address all correspondence to: sdas317@gmail.com

IntechOpen

References

[1] Murray NA, Roberts IAG. Haematology. In: Rennie JM, editor. Rennie & Robertson's Textbook of Neonatology. 5th ed. China: Elsevier Ltd; 2012. pp. 755-790

[2] Maheshwari A, Carlo WA. Hemolytic disease of the Newborn (erythroblastosis fetalis). In: Kliegman RM, Stanton BF, Schor NF, St Geme JW III, Behrman RE, editors. Nelson Textbook of Pediatrics. 19th ed. New Delhi: Thomas Press India Ltd; 2012. pp. 615-619

[3] Maitra A. Disease of infancy and childhood. In: Kumar V, Abbas AK, Fausto N, Aster JC, editors. Robbins and Cortan Pathologic Basis of Disease. 8th ed. New Delhi: Elsevier Inc.; 2010. pp. 447-486

[4] Kennedy MS. Perinatal issues in transfusion practices. In: Roback JD, Grossman BJ, Harris T, Hillyer CD, editors. Technical Manual. 17th ed. Maryland, United States: AABB; 2011. pp. 631-645

[5] Poole J, Daniels G. Blood group antibodies and their significance in transfusion medicine. Transfusion Medicine Reviews. 2007;**21**(1):58-71

[6] Klein HG, Anstee DJ, editors. Hemolytic disease of the fetus and the newborn. In: Mollison's Blood Transfusion in Clinical Medicine. 12th ed. Blackwell Scientific; 2014. pp. 499-549

[7] Koelewijn JM, Van Der Schoot CE, Bonsel GJ, De Haas M. Effect of screening for red cell antibodies, other than anti-D, to detect hemolytic disease of fetus and newborn: A population study in the Netherlands. Transfusion. 2008;**48**:941-952

[8] Moise KJJ. Hemolytic disease of the fetus and newborn. In: Creasy RK, Resnik R, Iams DJ, Lockwood CJ, Moore TR, Greene MF, editors. Creasy and Resnik's Maternal-Fetal Medicine: Principles and Practice. 2014

[9] Bowman J. Thirty-five years of Rh prophylaxis. Transfusion. 2003;**43**: 1661-1666

[10] Landsteiner K, Weiner A. An agglutinable factor in human blood recognized by immune sera for rhesus blood. Proceedings of the Society for Experimental Biology and Medicine. 1940;**43**:223-229

[11] Levine P, Katzin E, Burham L. Isoimmunization in pregnancy: Its possible bearing on the etiology of erythroblastosis fetalis. Journal of the American Medical Association. 1941;**116**:825-827

[12] Keenan H, Pearse W. Transplacental transmission of fetal erythrocytes. American Journal of Obstetrics & Gynecology. 1963;**86**:1096

[13] Liley A. Intrauterine transfusion of fetus in haemolytic disease. British Medical Journal. 1963;**2**:1107

[14] Wallerstein H. Treatment of severe erythroblastosis by simultaneous removal and replacement of blood of the newborn infant. Science. 1946;**103**: 583-584

[15] Chown B. The place of early induction in the management of erythroblastosis fetalis. Canadian Medical Association. 1958;**78**:252-256

[16] Finn R, Sheppard P, Lehane D, Kulke W. Experimental studies on the prevention of Rh hemolytic disease. British Medical Journal. 1961;**1486**:490

[17] Schneider JPO. Die profylaxe der thesis-sensibilisierung mit

Immunoglobulin anti-D. Ärztliche Forschung. 1967;**21**:11

[18] Kindt TJ, Goldsby RA, Osborne BA, editors. Antigens and Antibodies. In: Kuby Immunology. 6th ed. New York: W. H Freeman and Company; 2007. pp. 76-106

[19] Klein HG, Anstee DJ. Immunology of red cells. In: Klein HG, Anstee DJ, editors. Mollison's Blood Transfusion in Clinical Medicine. 12th ed. Wiley Blackwell; 2014. pp. 53-118

[20] Urbaniak J. Alloimmunity to human red blood cell antigens. Vox Sanguinis. 2002;**83**(Suppl. 1):293-297

[21] Brinc D, Lazarus AH. Mechanisms of anti-D action in the prevention of hemolytic disease of the fetus and newborn. Hematology American Society of Hematology. 2009:185-191

[22] Bowman J. RhD hemolytic disease of the newborn. The New England Journal of Medicine. 1998;**339**(24):1775-1777

[23] Kennedy MS. Hemolytic disease of the fetus and newborn (HDFN). In: Harmening D, editor. Modern Blood Banking & Transfusion Practices. 6th ed. New Delhi: Jaypee; 2013. pp. 427-438

[24] Egbor M, Knott P, Bhide A. Red-cell and platelet alloimmunisation in pregnancy. Best Practice & Research. Clinical Obstetrics & Gynaecology. 2012;**26**:112-132

[25] de Haas M, Thurik FF, Koelewijn JM, van der Schoot CE. Haemolytic disease of the fetus and the newborn. Vox Sanguinis. 2015;**109**:99-113

[26] Vaughan J, Manning M, Warwick RM, et al. Inhibition of erythroid progenitor cells by anti-Kell antibodies in fetal alloimmune anemia. The New England Journal of Medicine. 1998;**338**: 798-803

[27] Heathcote D, Carroll T, Flower R. Sixty years of antibodies to MNS system hybrid glycophorins: What have we learned? Transfusion Medicine Reviews. 2011;**25**:111-124

[28] Armstrong B, Smart E. Haemolytic diseases. International Society of Blood Transfusion Science Series. 2008;**3**: 93-109

[29] Klein HG, Anstee DJ, editors. The Rh blood group system (including LW and RHAG). In: Mollison's Blood Transfusion in Clinical Medicine. 12th ed. Oxford, UK: Wiley Blackwell; 2014. pp. 167-213

[30] Daniels G, editor. Rh and RHAG blood group system. In: Human Blood Groups. 3rd ed. Oxford, UK: Blackwell Scientific; 2013. pp. 182-258

[31] Sheeladevi CS, Suchitha S, Manjunath GV, Murthy S. Hemolytic disease of the newborn due to anti-c isoimmunization: A case report. Indian Journal of Hematology and Blood Transfusion. 2013;**29**(3):155-157

[32] Shastry S, Bhat S. Severe hemolytic disease of newborn in a Rh D-positive mother: Time to mandate the antenatal antibody screening. The Journal of Obstetrics and Gynecology of India. 2012:1-2

[33] Negi G, Singh GD. Anti Rh hemolytic disease due to anti C antibody: Is testing for anti D antibodies enough? Indian Journal of Hematology and Blood Transfusion. 2012;**28**(2): 121-122

[34] Chao A-S, Chao A, Ho S-Y, Chang Y-L, Lien R. Anti-E alloimmunization: A rare cause of severe fetal hemolytic disease resulting in pregnancy loss. Case Reports in Medicine. 2009;**2009**:1-2

[35] Ranasinghe E, Goodyear E, Burgess G. Anti-Ce complicating two consecutive pregnancies with increasing

severity of haemolytic disease of the newborn. Transfusion Medicine. 2003; **13**:53-56

[36] Moran P, Robson S, Reid M. Anti-E in pregnancy. British Journal of Obstetrics and Gynaecology;**107**: 1436-1438

[37] Joy SD, Rossi KQ, Krugh D, O'Shaughnessy RW. Management of pregnancies complicated by anti-E alloimmunization. The American College of Obstetricians and Gynecologists. 2005;**105**(1):24-28

[38] Chou ST, Westhoff CM. The Rh system. In: Roback JD, Grossman BJ, Harris T, Hillyer CD, editors. Technical Manual. 17th ed. Maryland, United States: AABB; 2011. pp. 389-410

[39] Whittle MJ. Rhesus haemolytic disease. Archives of Disease in Childhood. 1992;**67**:65-68

[40] Liumbruno GM, D'Alessandro A, Rea F, Piccinini V, Catalano L, Calizzani G, et al. The role of antenatal immunoprophylaxis in the prevention of maternal-foetal anti-Rh(D) alloimmunisation. Blood Transfusion. 2010;**8**:8-16

[41] Filbey D, Berseus O, Carlberg M. Occurrence of anti-D in RhD-positive mothers and the outcome of the newborns. Acta Obstetricia et Gynecologica Scandinavica. 1996;**75**: 585-587

[42] Prasad MR, Krugh D, Rossi KQ, O'Shaughnessy RW. Anti-D in Rh positive pregnancies. American Journal of Obstetrics and Gynecology. 2006; **195**(4):1158-1162

[43] Lacey PA, Caskey CR, Werner DJ, Moulds JJ. Fatal hemolytic disease of a newborn due to anti-D in an Rh-positive Du variant mother. Transfusion. 1983; **23**(2):91-94

[44] Wiener AS. A new test (blocking test) for Rh sensitization. Proceedings of the Society for Experimental Biology and Medicine. 1944;**56**:173-176

[45] Lee E. Blocked D phenomenon. Blood Transfusion. 2013;**11**:10-11

[46] Moiz B, Salman M, Kamran N, Shamsuddin N. Blocked D phenomenon. Transfusion. 2008;**48**(8):1545-1546

[47] Sulochana PV, Rajesh A, Mathai J, Sathyabhama S. Blocked D phenomenon, a rare condition with Rh D haemolytic disease of newborn-A case report. International Journal of Laboratory Hematology. 2008;**30**(3): 244-247

[48] Verma A, Sachan D, Bajpayee A, Elhence P, Dubey A, Pradhan M. RhD blocking phenomenon implicated in an immunohaematological diagnostic dilemma in a case of RhD-haemolytic disease of the foetus. Blood Transfusion. 2013;**11**(1):140-142

[49] Lee E, Redman M, Owen I. Blocking of fetal K antigens on cord red blood cells by maternal anti-K. Transfusion Medicine. 2009;**19**:139-140

[50] Gooch A, Parker J, British Committee for Standards in Haematology Blood Transfusion Task Force. Guideline for Blood Grouping and Antibody Testing in Pregnancy. 2007. pp. 252-262

[51] American College of Obstetricians and Gynecologists. ACOG practice bulletin No. 75: Management of alloimmunization during pregnancy. Obstetrics and Gynecology;**108**(2): 457-464

[52] Uhr J, Moller G. Regulatory effect of antibody on the immune response. Advances in Immunology. 1968;**8**:81-127

[53] Kumpel B, Elson C. Mechanism of anti-D-mediated immune suppression—A

paradox awaiting resolution? Trends in Immunology. 2001;**22**:26-31

[54] de Haas M, Finning K, Massey E, Roberts DJ. Anti-D prophylaxis: past, present and future. Transfusion Medicine. 2014;**24**(1):1-7

[55] Fung KFK, Eason E. Prevention of Rh Alloimmunization. SOGC Clin Pract Guidel. No. 133 2003. pp. 1-9

[56] Cohen DN, Johnson MS, Liang WH, McDaniel HL, Young PP. Clinically significant hemolytic disease of the newborn secondary to passive transfer of anti-D from maternal RhIG. Transfusion. 2014;**54**(11): 2863-2866

[57] Dean L. The Rh blood group. In: Blood Groups and Red Cell Antigens. Bethesda: National library of medicine (US), NCBI; 2006. pp. 1-6

[58] Hackney DN, Knudtson EJ, Rossi KQ, Krugh D, O'Shaughnessy RW. Management of pregnancies complicated by anti-c isoimmunization. The American College of Obstetricians and Gynecologists. 2004;**103**(1):24-30

[59] Rath MEA, Smits-Wintjens VEHJ, Walther FJ, Lopriore E. Hematological morbidity and management in neonates with hemolytic disease due to red cell alloimmunization. Early Human Development. 2011;**87**:583-588

[60] Allen F, Tippett P. A new Rh blood type which reveals the Rh antigen G. Vox Sanguinis. 1958;**3**:321-330

[61] Palfi M, Gunnarsson C. The frequency of anti-C + anti-G in the absence of anti-D in alloimmunized pregnancies. Transfusion Medicine. 2001;**11**:207-210

[62] Hadley A, Poole G, Poole J, et al. Haemolytic disease of the newborn due to anti-G. Vox Sanguinis. 1996;**71**: 108-112

[63] Vos G. The evaluation of specific anti-G (CD) eluate obtained by a double absorption and elution procedure. Vox Sanguinis. 1960;**5**:472-478

[64] Baía F, Muñiz-Diaz E, Boto N, Salgado M, Montero R, Ventura T, et al. A simple approach to confirm the presence of anti-D in sera with presumed anti-D+C specificity. Blood Transfusion. 2013;**11**(3):449-451

[65] Howard H, Martlew V, Mcfadyen I, Clarke C, Duguid J, Bromilow I, et al. Consequences for fetus and neonate of maternal red cell Allo-immunisation. Archives of Disease in Childhood Fetal and Neonatal Edition. 1998;**78**:62-66

[66] Nordvall M, Dziegiel M, Hegaard HK, Bidstrup M, Jonsbo F. Red blood cell antibodies in pregnancy and their clinical consequences : Synergistic effects of multiple specificities. Transfusion. 2009;**49**:2070-2075

[67] Kornstad L. New cases of irregular blood group antibodies other than anti-D in pregnancy. Frequency and clinical significance. Acta Obstetricia et Gynecologica Scandinavica. 1983;**62**(5): 431-436

[68] Chapman J, Waters A. Haemolytic disease of the newborn due to rhesus anti-e antibody. Vox Sanguinis. 1981; **41**(1):45-47

[69] Kollamparambil TG, Jani BR, Aldouri M, Soe A, Ducker DA. Anti-Cw alloimmunization presenting as hydrops fetalis. Acta Paediatrica. 2005;**94**:499-501

[70] Dajak S, Stefanović V, Capkun V. Severe hemolytic disease of fetus and newborn caused by red blood cell antibodies undetected at first-trimester screening. Transfusion. 2011;**51**(7): 1380-1388

[71] Fortner KB. The Johns Hopkins Manual of Gynecology and Obstetrics. 2007. p. 238

[72] Leger RM. Blood group terminology and the other blood groups. In: Harmening D, editor. Modern Blood Banking & Transfusion Practices. 6th ed. New Delhi: Jaypee; 2013. pp. 172-215

[73] Klein HG, Anstee DJ, editors. Other red cell antigens. In: Mollison's Blood Transfusion in Clinical Medicine. 12th ed. Oxford, UK: Wiley Blackwell; 2014. pp. 214-258

[74] Tovey L. Haemolytic disease of the newborn—The changing scene. British Journal of Obstetrics and Gynaecology. 1986;**93**:960-966

[75] Kamphuis MM, Lindenburg I, van Kamp IL, Meerman RH, Kanhai HHH, Oepkes D. Implementation of routine screening for Kell antibodies: Does it improve perinatal survival? Transfusion. 2008;**48**(5):953-957

[76] Grant S, Kilby M, Meer L, Weaver J, Gabra G, Whittle M. The outcome of pregnancy in Kell alloimmunisation. British Journal of Obstetrics and Gynaecology. 2000;**107**:481-485

[77] van Wamelen DJ, Klumper FJ, de Haas M, Meerman RH, van Kamp IL, Oepkes D. Obstetric history and antibody titer in estimating severity of Kell alloimmunization in pregnancy. Obstetrics and Gynecology. 2007;**109**(5):1093-1098

[78] Daniels G. Other blood groups. In: Roback JD, Grossman BJ, Harris T, Hillyer CD, editors. Technical Manual. 17th ed. Maryland, United States: AABB; 2011. pp. 411-436

[79] Kleinhauer K, Braun E, Betke K. Demonstration von fetalen haemoglobin in den erytrozyten eines blutausstrichs. Klin Wochenschr. 1957;**35**:637-640

[80] Caballero C, Vekemans M, Lopez del Campo J. Serum alpha-fetoprotein in adults, in women during pregnancy, in children at birth, and during the first week of life: A sex difference. American Journal of Obstetrics and Gynecology. 1977;**127**:384

[81] Seppala M, Ruoslahti E. Alpha fetoprotein in amniotic fluid: An index of gestational age. American Journal of Obstetrics and Gynecology. 1972;**114**: 595-598

[82] Fong EA, Davies JI, Grey DE, Reid PJ, Erber WN. Detection of massive transplacental haemorrhage by flow cytometry. Clinical and Laboratory Haematology. 2000;**22**(6):325-327

[83] de Haas M, Van der Schoot E. Prenatal screening. International Society of Blood Transfusion Science Series. 2013;**8**:6-10

[84] Bromilow IM, Adams KE, Hope J, Eggington JA, Duguid JK. Evaluation of the ID-gel test for antibody screening and identification. Transfusion Medicine. 1991;**1**(3):159-161

[85] Judd WJ. Practice guidelines for prenatal and perinatal immunohematology, revisited. Transfusion. 2001;**41**:1445-1452

[86] The Royal Australian and New Zealand College of Obstetricians and Gynaecologists. Guidelines for Blood Grouping and Antibody Screening in the Antenatal and Perinatal Setting. Aust New Zeal Soc Blood Transfus Ltd; 2007. pp. 1-24

[87] Minakami H, Maeda T, Fujii T, Hamada H, Iitsuka Y, Itakura A, et al. Guidelines for obstetrical practice in Japan: Japan Society of Obstetrics and Gynecology (JSOG) and Japan Association of Obstetricians and Gynecologists (JAOG) 2014 edition. The Journal of Obstetrics and Gynaecology Research. 2014;**40**(6):1469-1499

[88] Trudell KS. Detection and identification of antibodies. In: Harmening DM, editor. Modern Blood

Banking & Transfusion Practices. 6th ed. New Delhi: Jaypee; 2013. pp. 216-240

[89] Green RE, Klostermann DA. The Antiglobulin test. In: Harmening D, editor. Modern Blood Banking & Transfusion Practices. 6th ed. New Delhi: Jaypee; 2013. pp. 101-118

[90] Das S, Chaudhary R, Khetan D. A comparison of conventional tube test and gel technique in evaluation of direct antiglobulin test. Hematology. 2007;**12**: 175-178

[91] Nathalang O, Chuansumrit A, Prayoonwiwat W, Siripoonya P, Sriphaisal T. Comparison between the conventional tube technique and the gel technique in direct antiglobulin tests. Vox Sanguinis. 1997;**72**:169-171

[92] Novaretti M, Jens E, Pagliarini T, Bonifacio S, Dorlhiac-Llacer P, Chamone D. Comparison of conventional tube test technique and gel microcolumn assay for direct antiglobulin test: A large study. Journal of Clinical Laboratory Analysis. 2004;**18**:255-258

[93] Bajpai M, Kaur R, Gupta E. Automation in immunohematology. Asian Journal of Transfusion Science. 2012;**6**(2):140-144

[94] Weisbach V, Kohnhäuser T, Zimmermann R, Ringwald J, Strasser E, Zingsem J, et al. Comparison of the performance of microtube column systems and solid-phase systems and the tube low-ionic-strength solution additive indirect antiglobulin test in the detection of red cell alloantibodies. Transfusion Medicine. 2006;**16**:276-284

[95] Finck R, Lui-Deguzman C, Teng S-M, Davis R, Yuan S. Comparison of a gel microcolumn assay with the conventional tube test for red blood cell alloantibody titration. Transfusion. 2013;**53**(4):811-815

[96] Petz LD, Garratty G, editors. Hemolytic disease of Fetus and Newborn. In: Immune Hemolytic Anemia. United States of America: Elsevier; 1980. pp. 517-572

[97] Thakur MK, Marwaha N, Kumar P, Saha S, Thakral B, Sharma R, et al. Comparison of gel test and conventional tube test for antibody detection and titration in D-negative pregnant women: Study from a tertiary-care hospital in North India. Immunohematology. 2010; **26**(4):174-177

[98] Kurtz EM, Pappas AA, Cannon A. Laboratory identification of erythroblastosis fetalis. Annals of Clinical and Laboratory Science. 1982; **12**(5):388-397

[99] Liley A. Liquor amnii analysis in management of pregnancy complicated by rhesus immunization. American Journal of Obstetrics and Gynecology. 1961;**82**:1359

[100] Scott F, Chan FY. Assessment of the clinical usefulness of the "Queenan" chart versus the "Liley" chart in predicting severity of rhesus iso-immunization. Prenatal Diagnosis. 1998; **18**(11):1143-1148

[101] Divakaran TG, Waugh J, Clark TJ, Khan KS, Whittle MJ, Kilby MD. Noninvasive techniques to detect fetal anemia due to red blood cell alloimmunization: A systematic review. Obstetrics and Gynecology. 2001;**98**: 509-517

[102] Mari G. Middle cerebral artery peak systolic velocity: Is it the standard of care for the diagnosis of fetal anemia? Journal of Ultrasound in Medicine. 2005;**24**(5):697-702

[103] Papantoniou N, Sifakis S, Antsaklis A. Therapeutic management of fetal anemia : Review of standard practice and alternative treatment options. Journal of Perinatal Medicine. 2013;**41**: 71-82

[104] Schwartz J, Winters JL, Padmanabhan A, Balogun RA, Delaney

M, Linenberger ML, et al. Guidelines on the use of therapeutic apheresis in clinical practice—Evidence-based approach from the writing Committee of the American Society for apheresis: The sixth special issue. Journal of Clinical Apheresis. 2013;**28**:145-284

[105] Robinson A. Unsuccessful use of absorbed autologous plasma in Rh-incompatible pregnancy (letter). The New England Journal of Medicine. 1981; **305**:1346

[106] Yoshida Y, Yoshida H, Tatsumi K, et al. Successful antibody elimination in severe M-incompatible pregnancy. The New England Journal of Medicine. 1981; **305**:460-461

[107] Gottstein R, Cooke RWI. Systematic review of intravenous immunoglobulin in haemolytic disease of the newborn. 2003;6–11

[108] Morgan C, Cannell G, Addison R, et al. The effect of intravenous immunoglobulin on placental transfer of a platelet- specific antibody: Anti-PlA1. Transfusion Medicine. 1991;**1**:209-216

[109] Chitkara U, Bussel J, Alvarez M, Lynch L, Meisel R, Berkowitz R. High-dose intravenous gamma globulin: Does it have a role in the treatment of severe erythroblastosis fetalis? Obstetrics and Gynecology. 1990;**76**(4):703-708

[110] Santavy J. Hemolytic disease in the Newborn-history and prevention in the world and the Czech Republic. Biomedical Papers of the Medical Faculty of the University Palacky, Olomouc, Czech Republic. 2010;**154**(2): 147-151

[111] Oepkes D. The modern management of red cell alloimmunisation. Royal College of Obstetricians and Gynaecologists. 2003; **5**:15-20

[112] Rodeck C, Kemp J, Holman C, Whitmore D, Karnicki J, Austin M.

Direct intravascular fetal blood transfusion by fetoscopy in severe rhesus isoimmunisation. Lancet. 1981;**1**: 625-627

[113] Boulton F. Transfusion guidelines for neonates and older children. British Journal of Haematology. 2004;**124**(4): 433-453

[114] Phibbs RH, Francisco S. Advances in the theory and practice of exchange transfusions. California Medicine. 1966; **105**(6):442-453

[115] Li B, Jiang Y, Yuan F, Ye H. Exchange transfusion of least incompatible blood for severe hemolytic disease of the newborn due to anti-Rh17. Transfusion Medicine. 2010;**20**(1): 66-69

[116] Rath MEA, Lindenburg ITM, Brand A, Van Kamp IL, Oepkes D, Walther FJ. Exchange transfusions and top-up transfusions in neonates with Kell haemolytic disease compared to Rh D haemolytic disease. Vox Sanguinis. 2011;**100**:312-316

[117] Paediatrics AA. Management of hyperbilirubinemia in the newborn infant 35 or more weeks of gestation. Pediatrics. 2004;**114**: 297-316

[118] Green-top Guideline: The Management of Women with Red Cell Antibodies during Pregnancy. Royal College of Obstetricians and Gynaecologists; 2014. p 65

[119] Goodstein M. Neonatal red cell transfusion. In: Herman J, Manno C, editors. Pediatric Transfusion Therapy. Bethesda: AABB; 2002. p. 65

[120] Neonatal Jaundice. NICE Clin Guidel; 2010. p 98

[121] Avent ND. Antenatal genotyping of the blood groups of the Fetus. Vox Sanguinis. 1998;**74**:365-374

Section 2

Future Perspectives

A New Alternative Approach for RhD Incompatibility; Determination Fetal RhD Status via Biosensor Technology

Ebru Dündar Yenilmez, Umut Kökbaş and Abdullah Tuli

Abstract

Prenatal detection of the fetal RHD status in early stage of pregnancy is observed to be useful in the management of RhD incompatibility to identify fetuses at risk of hemolytic disease. The routine use of antenatal and postnatal anti-D prophylaxis reduces the incidence of hemolytic disease of the fetus and newborn. Cell-free fetal DNA in maternal plasma is in use today for routine genotyping fetal RHD status. Fetal RhD antigens can be detected in the blood of RhD-negative pregnant women using a nanopolymer-coated biosensor and could be an alternative method for medical diagnosis. We detected RhD-positive fetal antibodies with biosensor in maternal blood of RhD-negative mothers. The electrochemical measurements were performed on a PalmSens potentiostat and corundum ceramic-based screen-printed gold electrode. The demonstrated method has a different view for the detection of fetal RhD status in early pregnancy. The biosensor technology is useful and can be carried out rapidly in clinical diagnosis. Biosensors are also reproducible methods which give results quickly compared to noninvasive fetal RHD genotyping with real-time PCR-based techniques. We suggest that this method could become an alternative part of fetal RHD genotyping from maternal plasma as a prenatal screening in the management of RhD incompatibility.

Keywords: RhD incompatibility, fetal RhD, biosensor, hemolytic disease, RhD antigen

1. Introduction

The discovery of circulating fetal DNA by Lo et al. [1] has opened new possibilities for noninvasive prenatal diagnosis for investigators. It has been shown that this new source of fetal DNA also could be used for noninvasive prenatal determination of fetal RhD genotyping using the plasma of RhD-negative pregnant women [2]. RhD genotyping from maternal plasma is a valuable method to identify pregnancies that has a risk of hemolytic disease of the fetus and newborn (HDFN) [3].

The HDFN is caused by IgG antibodies of the mother that cross the placenta to red cell surface antigens and facilitate destruction to the immune defense of fetal red cells or erythroid progenitors. This causes a significant rate of morbidity and mortality for the fetus. RhD antigen of the rhesus system is the most commonly implicated antigen [4, 5]. Prophylaxis after delivery with anti-D immunoglobulin reduces the alloimmunization of RhD-negative women [4]. RhD alloimmunization has to be monitored for fetal anemia in complicated pregnancies for effective pre-/ postnatal transfusion treatment to prevent the baby from hydrops fetalis [3, 6].

Postnatal prophylaxis was used since the 1960s, with serology test used to identify the baby's RhD status [7]. The routine antenatal prophylaxis in the third trimester of pregnancy is now a standard implementation in many countries [4, 8, 9]. This application reduces the maternal sensitization and the HDFN in babies [7].

Invasive procedures should be avoided in alloimmunized pregnant women because of the risk of transplacental hemorrhage (amniocentesis has the risk up to 17%), and the risk of pregnancy loss was found to be up to 2% after amniocentesis and chorionic villous sampling (CVS), respectively [10].

In this chapter we aimed to share our experiences about the determination of fetal RhD genotyping with cffDNA and detection of fetal RhD antigens from maternal blood using a new biosensor as a candidate method for management of RhD incompatibility.

2. RhD incompatibility and management

The knowledge about the fetal RhD type supports the management of alloimmunized pregnancies in RhD-negative women [11, 12].

Prophylaxis after delivery is offered only to RhD-negative women who have given birth to an RhD-positive baby [9, 13]. This prevents babies from rhesus disease and reduces maternal sensitization. Routine antenatal anti-D prophylaxis use was first introduced in the mid-1990s. The sensitization rates were then reported to reduce from 1.2% for the earlier policy to 0.28% [7]. Commonly in white population, however, about 38% of these women would be carrying an RhD-negative fetus and thus receive anti-RhD immunoglobulin, a pooled human plasma product, unnecessarily [14, 15]. Fetal RHD genotyping with cell-free fetal DNA (cffDNA) is accepted as a useful method by obstetricians in early pregnancy for the management of RhD incompatibility. Since 2001, several European countries use cffDNA in maternal blood for noninvasive prenatal diagnosis of fetal RhD status [3]. There is also change in the measurement method in the hemolysis detection. This invasive method which detects the optical density at a wavelength of 450 nm in amnion fluid replaced by detect the fetal anemia by the Doppler measurement of the peak velocity of systolic blood flow in the middle cerebral artery [16].

3. Fetal RhD genotyping with cell-free fetal DNA

Prenatal care strategies for the fetus with RhD have been changed significantly during the last few decades. Discovered cffDNA from plasma of pregnant women by Lo et al., in 1997, has been used for the noninvasive detection of fetal RhD status which avoids RhD-negative women from antenatal anti-RhD prophylaxis [17–20].

3.1 Methods and sample preparation

3.1.1 Sample preparation

Maternal blood (10 cc) was collected from each pregnant woman and placed into an EDTA tube. Centrifugation step was applied within 1 h (at 1600 × g, 10 min) after separating maternal plasma. After centrifugation the plasma was removed carefully from the collection tubes and transferred into polypropylene tubes. Another centrifugation step was done at 16,000 × *g* (10 min). The plasma supernatants removed to new polypropylene tubes and stored at −20°C until other processes. Collected plasmas were thawed, and the DNA was automatically extracted from 1 mL of plasma as reported previously [9, 21, 22].

3.1.2 Fetal RhD genotyping

RHD genes (exons 5 and 7) were analyzed from isolated cffDNA samples. The oligonucleotide primers used to perform real-time quantitative PCR are reported in **Table 1** [9]. The gene of DYS14 was tested to confirm the presence of male fetal DNA, and the beta globin (β-globin) gene was used as a reference to confirm the presence of cffDNA [10]. Real-time PCR performed in a LightCycler 480 (Roche Applied Science, Basel, Switzerland) using 96-well plates. The PCR mixture was 50 μL in total volume that contains 300 nM of each primer, 50 nM probe, 2 × TaqMan Universal PCR master mix (Roche Diagnostics, Basel, Switzerland), and 15 μL of template DNA of plasma samples. The PCR cycling conditions were as follows. Incubation step was 50°C for 2 min and 95°C for 10 min. Amplification step was 95°C 15 s and 60°C 60 s (50 cycles). The β-globin gene protocol was the initialization step at 95°C for 10 min, followed by 95°C 15 s, 57°C 10 s, and 72°C 10 s (40 cycles). Samples were analyzed in triplicate. Calibration curves were run also for each analysis [21].

The clinical features of the subjects studied (mean age and week of pregnancy) are shown in **Table 2**. Fifteen fetuses were found to be RhD-negative females. The RhD status of the fetus was predicted in 70 pregnancies in our study. The gender determination of the fetuses was shown in **Table 3**.

We have shown that fetal RHD genotyping by multiplex real-time PCR is applicable and readily performed, with a high accuracy rate, as a routine clinical test in prenatal diagnostic laboratories in Turkey. This method avoids unnecessary

Primer	Sequence (5′–3′)	Label
RHD exon 7		
Forward	GGGTGTTGTAACCGAGTGCTG	None
Reverse	CCGGCTCCGACGGTATC	None
TaqMan probe	CCCACAGCTCCATCATGGGCTACAA	FAM-TAMRA
RHD exon 5		
Forward	CGCCCTCTTCTTGTGGATG	None
Reverse	GAACACGGCATTCTTCCTTTC	None
TaqMan probe	TCTGGCCAAGTTTCAACTCTGCTCTGCT	VIC-TAMRA
DYS14		
Forward	CATCCAGAGCGTCCC TGG	None
Reverse	TTCCCCTTTGTTCCCCAAA	None
TaqMan probe	CGAAGCCGAGCTGCCCATCA	FAM-TAMRA
Beta globin		
Forward	ACACAACTGTGT TCACTAGC	None
Reverse	CAACTTCATCCACGTTCACC	None
TaqMan probe	GAAGTCTGCCGTTACTGCCCTG	LC-Red

Table 1.
Primer and probe sequences used in RHD genotyping [9].

RhD status	Age (years)	Gestational age	Immunization	
	X ± SD (min–max)	X ± SD (min–max)	Yes (n, %)	No (n, %)
RhD-negative (n = 26)	29.1 ± 6.0 (20–39)	20.2 ± 8.6 (10–38)	12 (46.2)	14 (53.8)
RhD-positive (n = 44)	28.6 ± 6.1 (18–39)	16.9 ± 6.9 (9–38)	11 (25.0)	33 (75.0)

Table 2.
Clinical features of the study population [9].

Gestation weeks	N	RhD positive, n (%)		RhD negative, n (%)		Accuracy of *RHD* and sex genotyping, %
		Male	Female	Male	Female	
6–12	38	10	18	3	7	100
13–28	20	3	5	7	5	100
29–40	12	6	2	1	3	100
Subtotal		19	25	11	15	
Total	70	44 (62.8%)		26 (37.2%)		100

Table 3.
Fetal RhD and sex status of maternal plasma samples [9].

immunoprophylaxis in RhD-negative women bearing RhD-negative fetuses. We suggest that RHD genotyping should become an essential part of prenatal screening in the management of RhD incompatibility [9].

4. Biosensor in use to detect fetal RhD in maternal blood

Nowadays biosensors are universal devices which is used in biomedical diagnosis such as point-of-care monitoring of treatment and disease progression, drug discovery, forensics, and biomedical research [23]. They are widely used in different areas of healthcare [24]. The two main examples of biosensors are pregnancy tests and glucometers which are very successful devices. Biosensors have different transducing mechanisms based on signal generation (such as an electrochemical or optical signal) following the formation of antigen-antibody complexes [25]. Antibodies, enzymes, and synthetic biomolecules that are high-affinity reagents can be coupled to the transducer in order to provide specificity of the biosensors [23, 26].

We designed a new nanopolymer-coated electrochemical biosensor which is specific for the detection of fetal RhD antigens in the blood of pregnant women and results compared with cffDNA RHD genotyping with real-time PCR [26]. Biosensor technology is reproducible which can be used many times. The results can be generated quickly within a few minutes when compared to noninvasive fetal RHD genotyping with real-time PCR-based techniques. We suggest that biosensor technology could become a candidate method in early pregnancy in the management of RhD incompatibility.

4.1 Materials and methods

The bioelectrochemical measurements were performed with PalmSens potentiostat systems and gold working electrode combined with the auxiliary Au/Pd (98/2%) electrode and the reference Ag/AgCl electrode. Thermostatic working cell, magnetic stirrer, automatic pipets, and Milli-Q ultrapure water were used in the experiments.

4.1.1 Preparation procedure of the Au electrode surface

Cleaning electrode. First off all, the base of the working electrode surface was polished with alumina. And then the polished working electrode was sonicated in pure ethanol and Milli-Q ultrapure water for 10 min for removing undesired absorbable particles, respectively. For the last step of the electrode cleaning, five successive cyclic voltammogram sweeps were taken with bare working electrode between -1.0 and $+1.0$ V in 0.1 M HNO_3 solution.

RhD antibody immobilization onto Au electrode surface. Poly(Hema-Mac) nanopolymer was immobilized on the clean electrode's surface at room temperature via anilin (20 µL anilin and 20 µL RhD antibody). For trapping the antibody, a cross-linking agent (2.5% glutaraldehyde) was used. The modified working electrode was cleaned with Milli-Q ultrapure water for removing unbinding materials.

Principle of the electrobiochemical measurement. The measurement is based on the oxidation-reduction reactions of the RhD antibodies. All the measurements performed with thermostatic reaction cell included phosphate buffer (50 mM, pH 7.0) and potassium ferrocyanide [$K_4Fe(CN)_6$] as mediator complex, at 35°C. The charge transfer capacitance (electrochemical potential difference) of antigen-antibody interaction difference was measured by biosensor system (**Figure 1**).

Preparation of the samples. The working group has 26 RhD-negative primigravidas. All of them were admitted to the Department of Gynecology and Obstetrics and to the Department of Medical Biochemistry for prenatal diagnosis in different gestational ages (8th–36th weeks) that were analyzed in biosensor study for RhD status (**Table 4**). Written informed consent that was approved by the Ethics Committee of the Faculty of Medicine of Cukurova University was obtained from each subject. Blood samples were collected at ethylenediaminetetraacetic acid (EDTA) tube (Becton Dickinson, Bangkok, Thailand). Blood group test was identified by the Blood Bank Centre using slide/tube agglutination test, which includes antibodies against red blood cell antigens.

4.2 RhD antibody immobilization

UV polymerization of anilin was used for RhD antibody immobilization. Anilin's reduction potential is reducing at the UV light. A reversible manner was showed on the uncovered working electrode of the cyclic voltammogram of redox probe $Fe(CN)_6^{4-}/^{3-}$ (**Figure 2**). To inhibit the charge transfer among redox probe in solution on the Au electrode, a bioactive layer was applied on the surface of the electrode. The reversible behavior of the cyclic voltammograms turned into a capacitive shape (**Figure 2**).

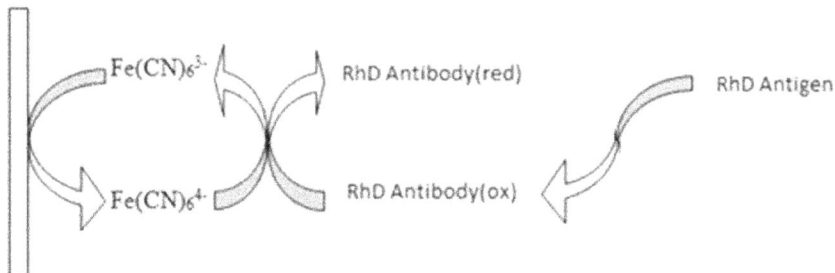

Figure 1.
The principle of the biosensor [26].

Fetal RhD Status	Age (years)		Gestational Age		Immunization
	X ± SD (min-max)	Range	X ± SD (min-max)	Range	
RhD positive (n = 21)	29.5 ± 5.9 (19–37)	18	15.1 ± 6.7 (8–36)	28	No
RhD negative (n = 5)	25.6 ± 3.2 (21–30)	9	11 ± 2.0 (8–13)	5	No

Table 4.
Clinical features of the samples in biosensor study for RhD status [26].

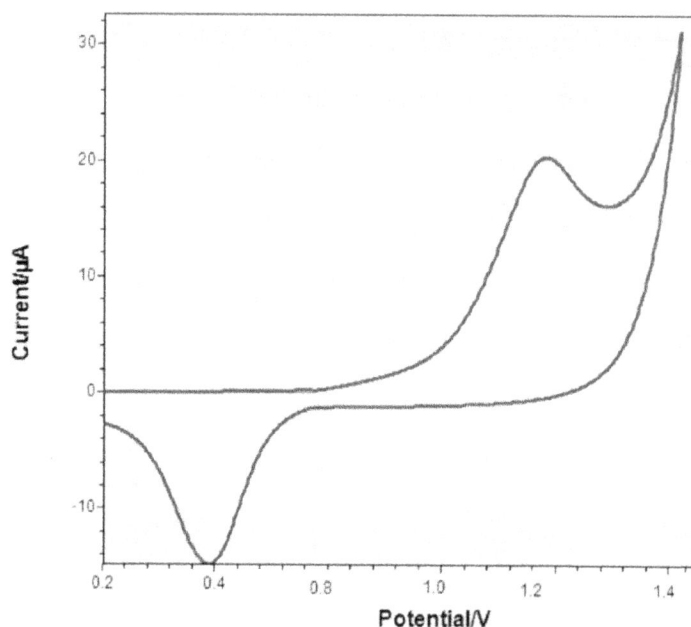

Figure 2.
RhD biosensors cyclic voltammogram for the immobilization steps. Red line: uncovered gold electrode; blue line: UV polymerized. (Working conditions: incubation time 1 h for RhD antibody; 50 mM electrochemical redox probe solution; and mediator complex pH 7.0 potassium ferrocyanide [$K_4Fe(CN)_6$]). For detection of RhD antigen in maternal sample, the optimal curve of the biosensors potential range was 0.2–1.4 V [26].

4.3 Biosensors optimization trials

Working condition optimization studies were performed to determine the most suitable working conditions for using the biosensor. For this aim, the mediator concentration, cross-linker concentration, RhD antibody concentration, temperature effect, pH, and repeatability were studied.

Concentration of RhD antibody. Determination of the antibody concentration effect on the biosensor response, different RhD antibody concentrations (0.05, 0.10, 0.15, 0.20 ng/mL) were applied on the surface of biosensor. The RhD antibodies optimum concentration was determined at 0.10 ng/mL.

Mediator and cross-linker concentration. In order to investigate the effect of the mediator concentration on the biosensor response, potassium ferrocyanide of 1.25 and 2.5 mg/dL was used in the preparation of the biosensor. To determine the effect of cross-linker concentration on the biosensor, the concentrations of glutaraldehyde of 12.5 and 2.5% were used. The optimum was value obtained at 2.5%. According to the results obtained from the experiments, the mediator complex of 1.25 mg/dL was assigned as the most effective result for the biosensor.

The pH effect. For the pH values' effect on the biosensor response, different buffer systems were investigated. For this aim, acetate (50 mM, pH 5.0 ± 5.5), phosphate (50 mM, pH 6.0 ± 6.5 ± 7.0 ± 7.5), and Tris-HCl (50 mM, 8.0 ± 8.5) buffers were used. The optimum pH value was found at 7.0 due to 100% activity rate. Above and below pH 7.0 can cause a decrease in the biosensor response.

Temperature effect. To examine the temperature effect on the biosensor response, the assay was performed by different temperatures (10 ± 55°C). The optimum working temperature of the biosensor system was detected as 35°C. The biosensor response is directly increased with temperature until 35°C, but further increase in temperature caused a decrease on the biosensor response.

Repeatability. Determination of the repeatability of the biosensor experiments were also studied for 1 μM RhD concentration (n = 10). From the assays the mean value ($\bar{x}$), standard deviation (SD), and coefficient of variation (CV %) were found to be 2.68 ± 0.06 μM and 2.23%, respectively. From the results, the repeatability of the biosensor response can be accepted as well as within the given concentration of RhD according to the 95% confidence interval.

4.4 Characterization of RhD antibody biosensor

The graphic shown as **Figure 3** is the concentrations of RhD in different gestational age of pregnant women. The slope of the curves increased with the increasing fetal RhD antigen concentration which depends on gestational ages of the samples (**Figure 3**).

Linearity. The linearity study for the RhD biosensor was obtained in concentration range between 1 and 250 ng/mL. At higher concentrations, standard curve showed a deviation from linearity.

Fetal RHD genotyping. The cffDNA used for fetal RhD status of the fetus is studied in 26 pregnancies with multiplex real-time PCR for RHD gene exons 5 and 7. Twenty-one of 26 cffDNA were detected as RhD positive, and 5 of 26 were detected as RhD negative (the same results as detection with RhD biosensor). The results of the fetuses were confirmed after the delivery by serological and molecular tests.

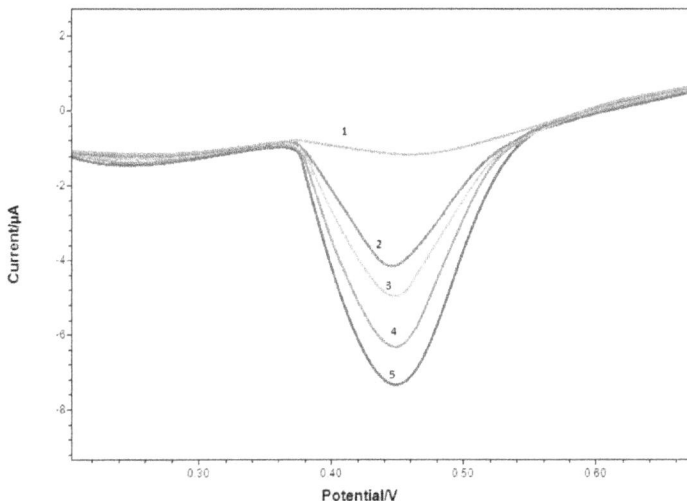

Figure 3.
Detection of increasing fetal RhD antigen with biosensor in different gestational age and mother's blood. Sloped line 1: RhD-negative sample; sloped line 2: sample 8th week of gestation; sloped line 3: sample 13th week of gestation; sloped line 4: sample 21th week of gestation; sloped line 5: sample 36th week of gestation [26].

5. Conclusions

The new biosensor design, which detects RhD status of the fetus in the early stage of pregnancy in RhD-negative pregnant women blood, is suggested as a candidate method in fetal RhD management. RhD antibody is immobilized using UV polymerization of anilin. To characterize the electrochemical properties of the biosensor surface, impedance measurements were applied. For binding the formed stable bioactive layer showed binding of RhD antigen of fetus. The significant impedance biosensor response concentration to detect RhD antigen-antibody binding was 1 ng/mL RhD. The fetus RhD status was approved with real-time PCR fetal RHD genotyping. The detection of the RhD status of the fetus with antigen-antibody biosensor system has more advantage as being fast compared to the noninvasive fetal *RHD* genotyping using fetal DNA. Up to now, common sero-logical-based techniques were used for the detection fetal RhD status on delivery. There is a requirement for fast, sensitive, and low-cost techniques on clinical and molecular diagnostic. Using NIPD for the fetal blood group, detection studies were accelerated after the discovery of fetal DNA in maternal plasma. The noninvasive technique of fetal RhD status of cffDNA with qPCR has been recently introduced and now is a strong alternative for traditional tests in early pregnancy. The early detection of RhD status with NIPD is advantageous and also avoids the mother from anti-RhD prophylaxis [5, 27]. For the detection of fetal *RHD* from maternal plasma, the fetal DNA extraction is a better way. In the last decade, there were significant improvements in the accurate management of pregnancies in RhD-negative preg-nant women (not immunized and/or alloimmunized) by noninvasive fetal *RHD* genotyping [12, 28].

The fetal nucleated red blood cells (RBCs) are well known in maternal blood [29]. Bianchi et al. disclosed that in the first three-month period of the gestation, the fetus blood contains plenty of RBCs [30]. The RBC membrane has the RhD antigen, and when the fetus genotype is RhD positive, the alloimmunization arise when the fetal RBCs enter maternal blood. The cause is the anti-D antibodies developed by RhD-negative mother. The fetal RhD antigens can be detected on the 30–40th day of pregnancy. During the measurement with biosensor, the fetal RhD antigens cause signals (the signals increased in proportion to the gestational week). This chemical signals mean that the fetal RhD antigens on fetal RBCs bind on the surface of the biosensor that is coated with RhD antibodies (antigen-antibody complex). In RhD-positive fetuses, this chemical signal is converted into an electrical signal by a transducer. In our RhD-negative samples (five of the fetus were RhD negative), there was no signal change detected on the biosensor. The biosensor detects the fetal RhD-positive antigens in the blood of RhD-negative mothers. This study demonstrates an original, quick, reliable, and easy detection method with biosensor technologies. The design of an immunospecific biosensor offers a candidate noninvasive prenatal detection for fetal RhD status to manage the RhD incompatibility between the fetus and mother. This method is able to capture fetal RhD antigens in maternal blood in the early stage of pregnancy (8th week of pregnancy). The biosensor-based detection of fetal RhD status takes several minutes using a gold electrode covered by RhD antibody. The determined biosensor method is more suitable, simple to construct, sensitive, and specific and does not require any expensive apparatus compared with the routine fetal RhD determination in early pregnancy. The biosensor instrument exhibits low cost with regard to real-time PCR devices. The biosensors can be used several times (up to 400-fold) and so decreases the cost. The most commonly used technique for NIPD is the qRT-PCR. Studies that based on biosensor technologies for NIPD applica-tion with cffDNA for monogenic diseases reported previously [31]. Some studies demonstrated PCR-free applications by SPR-imaging [32]. We prepared a study which detects fetal RHD genotypes from cffDNA using SPR-based biosensor.

In conclusion, the biosensor-based technologies which have used less amount of sample and low cost and determine the RhD status of the fetus in a very short time make the biosensors more advantageous than NIPD of RhD based on real-time quantitative PCR technologies.

Acknowledgements

We thank Cukurova University, Medicine Faculty, Obstetrics and Gynecology and Perinatology Department for sampling (chorionic villi) from mothers in first trimester.

Conflict of interest

There is no conflict of interest between authors.

Author details

Ebru Dündar Yenilmez*, Umut Kökbaş and Abdullah Tuli
Department of Medical Biochemistry, Faculty of Medicine, Cukurova University, Adana, Turkey

*Address all correspondence to: edundar@cu.edu.tr

IntechOpen

References

[1] Lo YMD, Corbetta N, Chamberlain PF, Rai V, Sargent IL, Redman CWG, et al. Presence of fetal DNA in maternal plasma and serum. The Lancet. 1997;**350**(9076):485-487

[2] Lo YM, Hjelm NM, Fidler C, Sargent IL, Murphy MF, Chamberlain PF, et al. Prenatal diagnosis of fetal RhD status by molecular analysis. New England Journal of Medicine. 1998;**339**:1734-1738

[3] Legler TJ, Muller SP, Haverkamp A, Grill S, Hahn S. Prenatal RhD testing: A review of studies published from 2006 to 2008. Transfusion Medicine and Hemotherapy. 2009;**36**(3):189-198

[4] Chitty LS, Finning K, Wade A, Soothill P, Martin B, Oxenford K, et al. Diagnostic accuracy of routine antenatal determination of fetal RHD status across gestation: Population based cohort study. BMJ. 2014;**349**:g5243

[5] Daniels G, Finning K, Martin P, Massey E. Noninvasive prenatal diagnosis of fetal blood group phenotypes: Current practice and future prospects. Prenatal Diagnosis. 2009;**29**(2):101-107

[6] van der Schoot CE, Hahn S, Chitty LS. Non-invasive prenatal diagnosis and determination of fetal Rh status. Seminars in Fetal and Neonatal Medicine. 2008

[7] Szczepura A, Osipenko L, Freeman K. A new fetal RHD genotyping test: Costs and benefits of mass testing to target antenatal anti-D prophylaxis in England and Wales. BMC Pregnancy and Childbirth. 2011;**11**(5)

[8] Clausen FB, Christiansen M, Steffensen R, Jørgensen S, Nielsen C, Jakobsen MA, et al. Report of the first nationally implemented clinical routine screening for fetal RHD in D−pregnant women to ascertain the requirement for antenatal RhD prophylaxis. Transfusion. 2012;**52**(4):752-758

[9] Yenilmez ED, Ozgünen FT, Evrüke IC, Tuli A. Noninvasive fetal RHD genotyping by multiplex real-time PCR in maternal plasma. International Journal of Current Medical Research. 2015;**4**(2):344-347

[10] Mujezinovic FAZ. Procedure-related complications of amniocentesis and chorionic villus sampling. Obstetrics & Gynecology. 2007;**110**(3):687-694

[11] Lo YMD, Bowell PJ, Selinger M, Mackenzie IZ, Chamberlain P, Gillmer MDG, et al. Prenatal determination of fetal RhD status by analysis of peripheral blood of rhesus negative mothers. The Lancet. 1993;**341**(8853):1147-1148

[12] Parchure DS, Kulkarni SS. Noninvasive fetal RHD genotyping from maternal plasma. Global Journal of Transfusion Medicine. 2016;**1**(1):21

[13] Benachi A, Delahaye S, Leticee N, Jouannic JM, Ville Y, Costa JM. Impact of non-invasive fetal RhD genotyping on management costs of rhesus-D negative patients: Results of a French pilot study. European Journal of Obstetrics, Gynecology, and Reproductive Biology. 2012;**162**(1):28-32

[14] Sbarsi I, Isernia P, Montanari L, Badulli C, Martinetti M, Salvaneschi L. Implementing non-invasive RHD genotyping on cell-free foetal DNA from maternal plasma: The Pavia experience. Blood Transfusion. 2012;**10**(1):34-38

[15] Ordonez E, Rueda L, Canadas MP, Fuster C, Cirigliano V. Evaluation of sample stability and automated DNA extraction for fetal sex determination using cell-free fetal DNA in maternal plasma. BioMed Research International. 2013;**2013**:195363

[16] Oepkes D, Seaward PG, Vandenbussche FP, Windrim R, Kingdom J, Beyene J, et al. Doppler ultrasonography versus amniocentesis to predict fetal anemia. New England Journal of Medicine. 2006;**355**(2):156-164

[17] Avent ND, Reid ME. The Rh blood group system: A review. Blood. 2000;**95**(2):375-387

[18] Lo YM. Recent developments in fetal nucleic acids in maternal plasma: implications to noninvasive prenatal fetal blood group genotyping. Transfusion Clinique et Biologique. 2006;**13**(1-2):50-52

[19] Van der Schoot CE, Soussan AA, Koelewijn J, Bonsel G, Paget-Christiaens LGC, de Haas M. Non-invasive antenatal RHD typing. Transfusion Clinique et Biologique. 2006;**13**(1-2):53-57

[20] Boggione C, Luján BM, Mattaloni S, Di Mónaco R, García BS, Biondi C, et al. Genotyping approach for non-invasive foetal RHD detection in an admixed population. Blood Transfusion;**2016**:1-8

[21] Yenilmez ED, Tuli A, Evruke IC. Noninvasive prenatal diagnosis experience in the Cukurova Region of Southern Turkey: Detecting paternal mutations of sickle cell anemia and beta-thalassemia in cell-free fetal DNA using high-resolution melting analysis. Prenatal Diagnosis. 2013;**33**(11):1054-1062

[22] Yenilmez ED, Tuli A. A non-invasive prenatal diagnosis method: Free fetal DNA in maternal plasma. Archives Medical Review Journal. 2013;**22**(3):317-334

[23] Bhalla N, Jolly P, Formisano N, Estrela P. Introduction to biosensors. Essays in Biochemistry. 2016;**60**(1):1-8

[24] Akkaya A, Altug C, Pazarlioglu NK, Dinckaya E. Determination of 5-aminosalicylic acid by catalase-peroxidase based biosensor. Electroanalysis. 2009;**21**(16):1805-1810

[25] Moina C, Gabriel Y. Fundamentals and applications of immunosensors. In: Chiu DNHL, editor. Advances in Immunoassay Technology. InTech; 2012. pp. 65-80

[26] Dundar Yenilmez E, Kokbas U, Kartlasmis K, Kayrin L, Tuli A. A new biosensor for noninvasive determination of fetal RHD status in maternal blood of RhD negative pregnant women. PloS one. 2018;**13**(6):e0197855

[27] Muller SP, Bartels I, Stein W, Emons G, Gutensohn K, Kohler M, et al. The determination of the fetal D status from maternal plasma for decision making on Rh prophylaxis is feasible. Transfusion. 2008;**48**(11):2292-2301

[28] Oxenford K, Silcock C, Hill M, Chitty L. Routine testing of fetal Rhesus D status in Rhesus D negative women using cell-free fetal DNA: An investigation into the preferences and information needs of women. Prenatal Diagnosis. 2013;**33**(7):688-694

[29] Sohda S, Arinami T, Hamada H, Nakauchi H, Hamaguchi H, Kubo T. The proportion of fetal nucleated red blood cells in maternal blood: Stimation by FACS analysis. Prenatal Diagnosis. 1997;**17**(8):743-752

[30] Bianchi DW. Fetal cells in the maternal circulation: Feasibility for prenatal diagnosis. British Journal of Haematology. 1999;**105**:574-583

[31] Feriotto G, Breveglieri G, Finotti A, Gardenghi S, Gambari R. Real-time multiplex analysis of four beta-thalassemia mutations employing surface plasmon resonance and biosensor technology. Laboratory Investigation. 2004;**84**(6):796-803

[32] Brouard D, Ratelle O, Perreault J, Boudreau D, St-Louis M. PCR-free blood group genotyping using a nanobiosensor. Vox Sanguinis. 2015;**108**(2):197-204

Chapter 5

ABO Blood Group Antigens as a Model of Studying Protein-Protein Interactions

Frida N. Gylmiyarova, Elena Ryskina, Nataliya Kolotyeva, Valeriia Kuzmicheva and Oksana Gusyakova

Abstract

This work presents a research of intermolecular interactions on the example of the antigen antibody interactions of the ABO system. This model could be successfully used in the future due to the lack of knowledge in the area of the ABO antigen's behavior as a biomolecule and the integration of these structures into chain of metabolic processes in a human being. Using computer PASS system ("in silico" research), we describe the possible biological effects of pyruvate, lactate, and antigen determinants A and B. Glycoproteins A and B are very perspective to study as biological active connectors due to the wide range of their biological effects. The obtained knowledge proves that ABO antigen, as well as other glycoprotein conjugates, could play an important role in intercellular adhesion and signal transmission, which could be used in perspective in personalized medicine, target therapy, and evaluation of lab results in clinical practice.

Keywords: ABO blood groups, protein-protein interaction, computer modeling, biological activity

1. Introduction

Erythrocytes are the most common blood cells in the human body. They present on their surface a huge number of different receptors and antigens, which explain their multiple biological functions. Since 1900, when Carl Landsteiner first found red blood cell antigens and named them ABO blood group system, a big step forward was made by scientists in this direction. Up to now, over 35 blood groups are registered in the International Society of Blood Transfusion. Some of them as ABO blood groups, MNS, Rh, Lutheran, Kell, Lewis, and Duffy are well studied and found their place in clinical practice, but others as Ok, Scianna, Colton, and Knops are on their way to be fully understood. The genes of the blood groups are mainly autosomal with the exception of XG, XK, and MIC2 genes as they are presented on X and Y chromosomes.

The biochemical structure of blood group antigens differs a lot; they can either be proteins (Rh, Kell) or glycoproteins and glycolipids (ABO) [1].

ABO blood group system consists of three alleles, dominant A and B, and recessive O, and it is controlled by a gene located on chromosome 9 (9q34.2).

These genes (A and B) code different glycosyltransferases: glycosyltransferase A which adds N-acetylgalactosamine and glycosyltransferase B which adds D-galactose to H-substance. O allele is inactive and does not encode an enzyme, so that H substance remains unmodified with a fucose moiety. Combinations of these three alleles give us four different blood groups O (I), A (II), B (III), and AB (IV) [2].

It is notable that ABO antigens are expressed not only on the surface of erythrocyte, but they can also be found in a variety of tissues and cells, such as the endothelium of blood vessels, neurons, epithelium, platelets, etc.

In recent years, the amount of research on protein-small molecule (metabolite) interactions has increased significantly. However, the study of these interactions, according to the 2011 Wiley Online Library, is lagging far behind other types of interactions, such as protein-protein, protein-DNA, and protein-RNA, in terms of publications. Only in 2009 the first publications about protein-metabolite interactions appeared.

From a biochemical point of view, most biological systems work by fulfilling their diverse functions by proteins. Due to the revolutionary progress in the study of genomics and proteomics, a more accurate idea of the amount of proteins synthesized in the body has now been formed, but there is a weak idea of which proteins nonspecifically interact with metabolites [3].

It has been established that intermolecular interactions play a crucial role in almost all major biological processes, such as cell regulation, biosynthesis and biodegradation, signal transmission, transcription and translation processes, the formation of oligomers and multimolecular complexes, packaging of viruses, and the immune response, are protein-ligand interactions [4]. The polyfunctionality of proteins is due to their ability to change the conformation of a molecule when interacting with ligands. Proteins can interact with almost all types of molecules: from small compounds—water, metal ions, carbohydrates, fatty acids, and cell membrane phospholipids—to high molecular weight proteins and nucleic acids. Disruption of protein interactions underlies some diseases [5].

This fact provides a key argument that biological and clinical significance of blood groups in general and ABO especially extends far beyond our expectations and needs to be clarified.

2. Computer modeling of antigen determinants A and B

2.1 Antigen A and its predicted biological activity

It is almost impossible to evaluate the specific properties of the terminal fragments of antigenic structures in an experiment, but with the method of computer simulation, one can predict the biological effects of substances.

Glycosylation of protein molecules significantly affects their ability to contact with other molecules, which is important for understanding the mechanisms of intermolecular interactions, signaling, and adhesion at the cellular and molecular levels. The group-specific antigens of the blood ABO system are formed by the glycosylation of transmembrane proteins presented on the surface of red blood cells.

A-Antigen terminal monosaccharide N-acetylgalactosamine contains in the position C2 NHCOCH3 group, and B-antigen terminal monosaccharide D-galactose, in position C2, contains OH group. Functional groups confer variability in the structure of antigens and provide specificity for binding ligands. The presence in the structure of the N-acetylgalactosamine acetyl group leads to the disappearance of the positive charge.

N-Acetylgalactosamine is an amino sugar found in almost all glycoproteins. The immediate precursor of N-acetylgalactosamine is fructose-6-phosphate. Amino sugar is further acetylated with acetyl-CoA.

Monosaccharides can take part in all reactions which are typical for hydroxyl-containing compounds: they form esters and ethers, acetals and ketals, undergo substitution and elimination reactions. An important property of monosaccharides is their ability to form glycosides due to hydroxyl at the first carbon atom. Elucidation of the potential biological activity of antigens, determined by the structural characteristic of the antigenic determinants of the ABO system, is an important task.

We used a program for computer modeling called PASS. Prediction of Activity Spectra for Substances (PASS) is a program designed for computer modeling created by a group of Russian scientists. This tool is based on the dependence between chemical formula of a random substance and its functional activity. Chemical formula is described using Multilevel Neighborhoods of Atom (MNA) descriptors, the combination of which is unique for each substance. The user gets the list of probable activities based on the program's self-educating "training set," which aggregates data on active compounds from databases, publications, and patents, marked with Pa (probability to be active) and Pi (probability to be inactive), placed in the order from the maximum Pa to the minimum one. The program uses the Bayesian approach with some modifications for calculating the Pa and Pi (for more detailed information, see [6, 7]). In our study we chose effects with Pa >0.5. Total number of biological activities in the database is 4130, 501 of them are pharmacological effects, 3295 are molecular mechanisms of action, 57 are toxic effects, 199 are mediated metabolic actions, and 29 are influences on gene expression.

We have identified a significant number of previously unknown properties and mechanisms of action for the antigenic determinant antigen A, namely, 99 out of 501 possible pharmacological effects, 304 out of 3295 possible molecular mechanisms of action, 17 out of 57 adverse and toxic effects, 12 of 199 metabolic-related activities, 2 of 29 effects regulating the expression of genes, and 5 of 49 effects associated with the transport of substances. We chose biological activities with a probability of Pa greater than 0.5. The PASS program allowed us to establish that the antigenic determinant of antigen A exhibits the following pharmacological effects (**Table 1**).

It is predicted that the antigenic determinant of antigen A exhibits antibacterial, immunostimulating, antifungal, antiviral, and pharmacological effects, as well as antibiotic properties.

Pharmacological effect	Pa	Pi	Pa − Pi
Membrane permeability agonist	0.840	0.006	0.834
Antibacterial	0.707	0.005	0.702
Immunostimulating	0.697	0.07	0.690
Antineoplastic	0.654	0.016	0.638
Antifungal	0.632	0.013	0.619
Antiviral	0.620	0.011	0.609
Angiogenesis stimulator	0.577	0.012	0.565
Vasoprotector	0.552	0.045	0.507

Table 1.
Predicted pharmacological effects of antigen A.

ABO phenotypic analysis of blood groups is often used to detect the degree of susceptibility of a person to infectious diseases. In the literature, there are data in which it is noted that the interaction of certain parasites and bacteria with human cells depends on the presence of certain blood groups [8].

Thus, antigen A exhibits high adhesive activity against lactic acid bacteria. Some of the antigens affect the humoral and cellular response [9].

For the oligosaccharide of the antigen A, the antineoplastic effect on the cancer of various etiologies and localization is predicted: gastric and lung cancer, sarcoma, leukemia, and cancer of the brain and ovaries. Numerous studies have shown an association between ABO blood groups and the risk of developing various types of cancer [10].

With a high degree of probability, the antigen A is able to regulate angiogenesis and has a potential vasoprotective effect, as well as an effect of inhibitor of membrane permeability and integrity. The formation of new blood vessels in the organ or tissue is activated only when the damaged tissues are regenerated. Some factors, depending on the dose, can be both inducers of angiogenesis and inhibitors [11]. Many predicted effects of the antigenic determinant of antigen A are realized through the molecular mechanisms of its action (**Table 2**).

It is predicted that the oligosaccharide of the antigen A can act as an agonist of nerve growth factor, tumor necrosis factor, hyaluronic acid, α-interferon, interleukin-2, and tissue kallikrein inhibitor. The stimulating effect of the oligosaccharide antigen A on the activity of caspases 3, 8, and 9, participants in the apoptosis process, is predicted. As it is known, all caspases are synthesized in an inactive form and are activated when necessary by initiating caspases in the process of partial proteolysis. Probably, the antigenic determinant A, by activating caspases, can trigger a signal chain of programmed cell death.

Analyzing molecular mechanisms of action of antigenic determinants A, we paid attention to the inhibitory effect, to a number of carbohydrate metabolism enzymes, complex lipid metabolism, and protein biosynthesis process.

Molecular mechanism of action	Pa	Pi	Pa − Pi
Inhibitor of CDP-glycerol phosphotransferase	0.837	0.006	0.931
A-glucosidase inhibitor	0.826	0.001	0.825
Analogue of insulin	0.755	0.003	0.552
Antagonist of membrane integrity	0.731	0.009	0.713
Lactase inhibitor	0.718	0.007	0.711
Nerve growth factor agonist	0.715	0.007	0.708
Inhibitor ceramide glycosyltransferase	0.713	0.010	0.703
Aspartyl transferase inhibitor	0.708	0.007	0.701
Hyaluronic acid agonist	0.701	0.002	0.699
B-glucuronidase inhibitor	0.661	0.005	0.656
Caspase stimulator	0.646	0.005	0.641
N-acetylglucosamine transferase inhibitor	0.636	0.003	0.633
Glycerol monooxidase inhibitor	0.628	0.025	0.603
A-interferon agonist	0.595	0.019	0.576
TNF agonist	0.550	0.019	0.531
IL-2 agonist	0.517	0.011	0.503

Table 2.
Predicted molecular mechanisms of action of antigen A.

Oligosaccharide antigen A may inhibit the activity of enzymes involved in the metabolism of simple carbohydrates, such as α-glucosidase, β-glucuronidase, and β-galactosidase, and in the exchange of complex carbohydrates, predominantly heteropolysaccharides—α-N-acetyl-glucosaminidase, dolichol glycosyltransferase, and GDP-mannose-6-dehydrogenase, which creates the possibility of inhibiting the metabolism of the components of the extracellular matrix of connective tissue—glycoproteins and proteoglycans. Dolichol glycosyltransferase plays a leading role in the glycosylation of membrane proteins.

It is predicted that the oligosaccharide of the antigen A can be an agonist of hyaluronic acid. Hyaluronic acid belongs to the innate immunity system and is involved in tissue regeneration, as evidenced by the likely manifestation of the pharmacological effects of tetrasaccharide A, as immunostimulating and vasoprotective.

Also, we predicted possible toxic effects (**Table 3**).

The effect of carbohydrate determinants of antigen A on the metabolism of complex lipids is predicted, and the molecular mechanism of action is inhibition of the activity of CDP-glycerol glycerophosphotransferase, ceramide glycosyltransferases, ganglioside galactosyltransferases, and galactosylglucosylceramidase, involved in the synthesis of phospho- and glycolipids, necessary for the construction of cell membrane structures. Glycolipids play an important role in making cell-to-cell contacts; some serve as a kind of receptor for a number of bacterial toxins.

The possibility of an inhibitory effect on a gene expressing telomerase was predicted. About 85% of cancer cells acquire unlimited replicative potential due to the reactivation of a specific telomerase enzyme [12].

After analyzing the data obtained by computer prediction, we can conclude that the immunochemical specificity of the antigenic determinant of antigen A is realized by the characteristic and diverse biological activity and toxicity.

2.2 Antigen B and its biological activity

The antigenic determinant of antigen B contains terminal D-galactose, at position C2 where it has a hydroxyl group.

D-Galactose itself can enter into the reactions of alkylation, acylation, reduction, and oxidation. Analysis of the data of the probable biological activities of the antigenic determinant of antigen B showed 106 out of 501 possible pharmacological effects, 311 of the 3295 probable molecular mechanisms of action, 16 of 57 adverse and toxic effects, 15 of 199 metabolically mediated actions, 3 of 29 effects regulating gene expression, and 6 of 49 effects associated with transport of substances. We chose biological activities with a probability of Pa greater than 0.5. The pharmacological effects of the antigenic determinant of antigen B are shown in **Table 4**.

Toxic effects	Pa	Pi	Pa − Pi
Hypokalemia	0.744	0.033	0.711
Nephrotoxicity	0.734	0.018	0.716
General toxicity	0.691	0.038	0.653
Bronchoconstrictor	0.647	0.035	0.612
Cardiotoxicity	0.644	0.031	0.613
Hepatotoxicity	0.611	0.051	0.560
Embryotoxic	0.504	0.012	0.492

Table 3.
Possible toxic effects of antigen A.

Pharmacological mechanism	Pa	Pi	Pa − Pi
Agonist of membrane permeability	0.863	0.005	0.858
Antibacterial	0.688	0.05	0.683
Immunostimulatory	0.668	0.008	0.660
Antineoplastic	0.630	0.021	0.609
Antifungal	0.622	0.014	0.608
Vasoprotector	0.599	0.042	0.557
Angiogenesis activator	0.591	0.010	0.581
Antiviral	0.583	0.014	0.569
Antibiotic	0.524	0.005	0.519

Table 4.
Predicted pharmacological effects of antigen B.

Many effects and mechanisms of action are common for both antigen A and antigen B, but they are characterized by different degrees of probability of manifestation (Pa value). It is predicted that the antigen B is able to exhibit antibacterial, antiviral, antifungal, and pharmacological effects. According to the literature, group-specific antigens A and B can play a direct role in the susceptibility of the infection, acting as receptors or co-receptors for microorganisms, parasites, and viruses (**Table 5**).

In the study, Kato shows that carbohydrates can act not only as receptors for various microbes but also function as a barrier to infection [13].

Numerous molecular mechanisms of the action of antigen B tetrasaccharide have been predicted, in particular the inhibitory effect on the activity of a number of enzymes involved in the metabolism and stimulating effects on various bioregulators.

Molecular mechanism of action	Pa	Pi	Pa − Pi
Inhibitor of CDP-glycerol phosphotransferase	0.806	0.008	0.798
A-glucosidase inhibitor	0.799	0.001	0.798
Antagonist of membrane integrity	0.764	0.010	0.754
Agonist of hyaluronic acid	0.720	0.001	0.719
Nerve growth factor agonist	0.701	0.009	0.709
Insulin agonist	0.699	0.004	0.695
Antagonist of interferon	0.603	0.017	0.586
Inhibitor of glycerol oxidase	0.638	0.023	0.615
Caspase 8 activator	0.625	0.007	0.618
TNF regulator	0.570	0.014	0.556
B-galactosidase inhibitor	0.558	0.003	0.555
IL-2 agonist	0.526	0.018	0.508
Caspase 3 activator	0.514	0.014	0.500
Glycosyltransferase inhibitor	0.512	0.004	0.508
Inhibitor of protein synthesis	0.509	0.007	0.502

Table 5.
Predicted molecular mechanisms of action of antigen B.

The stimulating effect of oligosaccharide B on the activity of caspases 3 and 8 is predicted; it can act as an agonist of hyaluronic acid, nerve growth factor, interleukin-2, and interferon antagonist. It has been established that galactooligo-saccharides selectively increase the content of useful intestinal microbes, as well as C-reactive protein and interleukins [14].

The probable effect of oligosaccharide B on the expression of the telomerase gene (Pa 0.785) and the transport of electrons in mitochondria (Ra 0.504) is shown. Oligosaccharide B is highly likely to be a substrate for cytochrome P-450 2J2 (Pa 0.980), glutathione-S-transferase (0.907), and cyclooxygenase (Pa 0.759).

Using PASS we also identified possible toxic effects (**Table 6**).

The PASS program revealed that the antigenic determinant of antigen B can exhibit a variety of biological effects and molecular mechanisms of action that regulate various physiological and metabolic processes in the body.

The role of carbohydrates as key biological ligands is well known. This is due to the high degree of isomerism, possible within individual carbohydrate units, in a variety of ways to combine monosaccharides, among themselves, different varia-tions of substituents (acetyl, sulfate) and flexibility of carbohydrate chains.

With the development of computational methods for studying protein-ligand interactions, it became possible to determine the type of bonds and the most important positions of atoms "C" in monosaccharides for the formation of an antigen-antibody complex. Using the molecular docking method, Stanca-Kaposta with a group of scien-tists found that hydrogen bonds and hydrophobic and van der Waals interactions are involved in the formation of an antigen-antibody association [15]. Monosaccharides of antigens can act as acceptors of hydrogen, and amino acid residues of paratope antibodies can serve as hydrogen donors. Most commonly, hydrogen bonds form atoms "C" at positions 3 and 5 in terminal galactose (antigen B) and atoms "C" at position 5 in N-acetylgalactosamine (antigen A). Accessibility of the nitrogen atom in the GalNAc epitope to participate in the formation hydrogen bonds are hampered by the presence of an acetyl group. The "C" atoms in position 6 are involved in hydrophobic and van der Waals interactions, both in galactose and in N-acetylgalactosamine [16].

In studies by J. Milland, it was found that in the N-acetylated version of the epit-ope of antigen A, the interaction of the acetyl group of the epitope with the tyrosine 35 of the immunoglobulin heavy chain precludes further penetration of the antigen into the antibody's binding site. In contrast, the Gal epitope of antigen B penetrates deeper into the antibody's binding site, and the second galactose antigenic determi-nant participates in hydrophobic interactions with tryptophan at position 36 of the immunoglobulin heavy chain [17]. ABO antigens, like other glycoconjugates, are important intercellular adhesion mediators and participants in signal transduction. Due to the diversity of biological effects manifested, oligosaccharides A and B are evaluated from a new perspective side as biologically active compounds and not only blood group antigens that protect blood cells [18].

Toxic effects	Pa	Pi	Pa − Pi
Hypokalemia	0.763	0.030	0.733
Nephrotoxicity	0.709	0.022	0.687
Bronchoconstrictor	0.703	0.026	0.677
Cardiotoxicity	0.687	0.023	0.664
General toxicity	0.667	0.043	0.624
Hepatotoxicity	0.590	0.057	0.533

Table 6.
Possible toxic effects of antigen B.

Computer modeling exists as a way of combining the microscopic world of molecules and experimental results, which helps to confirm our understanding of metabolic processes and propose new directions for research. For many of the predicted types of activity of compounds in the available literature, experimental evidence has not been found, since these organic compounds are difficult for conformational analysis. Computational methodology makes it possible to obtain structures of compounds at the atomic level and information about activity with an accuracy equivalent to or greater than can be obtained in an experiment. The prognostic and interpretative program PASS has helped to better present the mechanisms of action of the studied metabolites and carbohydrate determinants of antigens A and B in relation to the main body systems.

3. ABO system as a marker of metabolic state

We selected 3678 healthy people with no chronic somatic and dental diseases, as well as latent socially significant viral infections (hepatitis B and C, HIV). Then, we performed a complex biochemical testing of blood with 40 parameters, complete blood count with 21 parameters, and hemostasiograms with 8 parameters. Studies of concentration of total protein; albumin; immunoglobulins A, G, and M; urea; creatinine; uric acid; total and direct bilirubin; C-reactive protein; alanine amino-transferase; aspartate aminotransferase; gamma-glutamyltranspeptidase; creatine kinase and creatine kinase-MB fraction; total cholesterol content; triglycerides; high-density lipoprotein and low-density lipoprotein; lipase activity; the coefficient of atherogenicity; glucose concentration; lactate dehydrogenase; alpha-amylase; alkaline phosphatase activity; and magnesium, calcium, phosphorus, and iron levels were carried out on an automatic biochemical analyzer "Hitachi-902" and "Integra 800" ("Roche," Japan) with the help of a commercial reagent kit from the company "Roche" (Germany). Intra-laboratory quality control when performing studies was carried out using control serum Precinorm and Precipath (Roche, Germany).

Complete blood count was performed using an automated hematology analyzer Sysmex KX-21 (Roche, Japan) using a commercial set of reagents produced by Roche (Germany). We measured distribution curves for the size of erythrocytes, leukocytes, and platelets, as well as analytical results for 18 parameters: the number of erythrocytes, leukocytes, and platelets; the content of hemoglobin and hema-tocrit; the average volume of erythrocytes and platelets; the average content and average concentration of hemoglobin in the erythrocyte; the width of the distribu-tion of erythrocytes and platelets by volume; the relative and absolute content of neutrophils, medium cells, and lymphocytes; and the ratio of large platelets. The morphological study of blood cells was performed using a Zeiss light microscope using a unified method. The erythrocyte sedimentation rate was determined using a Panchenkov unified micromethod. The functionality of platelets was assessed by the method of visual detection of the start time of aggregation with different induc-tors (ADP, with a universal aggregation inducer (UIF), collagen).

Statistical processing of the results was carried out using the statistical pack-age SPSS 12.0 and Microsoft Excel 2007. The statistical characteristics were used: arithmetic average (M), standard arithmetic average error (m), median (Me), max, min, and 95% interval. Indicators of skewness and steepness reflect the asymmetry of distribution; normality tests were evaluated using the Kolmogorov-Smirnov test with the Lilyfors and Shapiro-Wilkie corrections. We used the nonparametric Mann-Whitney U test with the amendment of Bonferroni as an alternative to the Student's t-test. Taking into account the deviation from normality of various values of dispersions, a nonparametric analogue of dispersive analysis was used—the

Kruskal-Wallis analysis. To study the correlation of blood parameters, Spearman's correlation analysis was used.

The data we obtained supplemented information about the connection of certain diseases with blood groups (**Table 7**).

On the basis of the study of the metabolism in the O (I)—AB (IV) blood groups, we determined the trends characterizing their biological variability and identified the parameters associated with a specific blood group (**Table 8**).

According to the specifics of these indicators, we attributed the owners of AV (IV) blood groups to the protein type, since they have the highest protein availability and they are less likely to get ill. It is known that A (II) carriers of the second blood group suffer from a wide range of diseases, including infectious diseases. They have an immunological memory of old and fresh contacts with bacterial and viral agents. The level of lipids can be conditionally attributed to the lipid type. In the presence of the first blood group, a high level of specific and nonspecific protection factors is characteristic. For them, a preferential connection with somatic pathology has been identified. Owners of the third blood group are characterized by sufficient good health. They have the highest level of albumin, cholesterol [19].

The identified features of the metabolic profile in individuals with different blood groups are the rationale for the individualization of standards for each person. In the future, every citizen should have his own health passport.

In accordance with the results obtained, in persons with O (I) blood group, a lower number of erythrocytes are noted with a relatively small volume of cells.

Blood group	Possibility of pathological process development	Authors
O (I)	Peptic ulcer disease	U. Altuhov (1983); G. Drannik,
	Stomach cancer	G. Dizik (1990)
	Hip joint dysplasia	A. Tananyan (2001);
	Myasthenia	S. Garmonov et al. (2006)
	Mutation (F7)	Wang Qing-yun (2007);
	Women papillomavirus infection	Bogdanov N.N. (2015)
	Acute inflammatory processes in women	B. Bjorkholmet al (2001)
	reproductive system	M. Aspholm-Hurtig et al. (2006)
	Sympathetic ophthalmia	I. Taboridze (1991)
	Laryngeal cancer	B. Gehte (1996)
	HCV	T. Subbotina (2012)
	Risk factor for ovarian reserve	E. Shevchenko (2010)
	Hemophilic patients with anemia	L. Arkhipova (2012)
	Rare bleeding disorders	T. Jin et al. (2016)
	Rare intraductal papillary mucinous neoplasm	X. Li et al.(2016)
	Rare case of malaria	J. Deng (2016)
	Rare hepatocellular carcinoma	U. Kosyakova
	Rare postpartum blood loss	F. Gilmiarova
		L. Spieza (2018)
		K. Poruk (2018)
		A. Degarege (2018)
		F. Liu (2018)
		M. Kahr (2018)
	Chronic prostatitis with benign prostatic hyperplasia	Shatohin M., Konoplya A., Dolgareva C. A., (2011)
	Bladder cancer	Mayskov I., (2013)
	Urolithiasis	Gusein-zade, R., (2013)
	The increased spontaneous platelet aggregation	Gergesova E., (2011)
	CHD	Biswas S., Ghoshal P.K., Halder B., Mandal N. (2013)

Blood group	Possibility of pathological process development	Authors
A (II)	Coronary artery disease	Z. Chen et al. (2016)
	Rheumatic diseases	E. Suslova (2012)
	CHD	E. Meshalkin (1981)
	Bronchial asthma	M. Freidin et al. (2006)
	Allergies	M. Rafalovich et al. (1982)
	Cholecystitis, cholelithiasis	E. Chichenko, U. Koshel (1975)
	Diabetes mellitus	B. Geht et al.(1995)
	Meningococcal infection	G. Dizik et al.(1986)
	Secondary purulent meningitis	A. Veselov, N. Malushkina
	Leiden mutation (F5)	(1988)
	Prothrombin mutation (F2)	U. Rudometov et al. (1981)
	Platelet receptors mutation (GpIa, GpIIIa)	I. Danilov (2010)
	Thromboembolism	R. Vitkovskiy
	HIV	E. Gergesova (2011)
	The combined prevalence of HIV and hepatitis C	G. Liumbruno (2013)
	Hepatitis B	S. Vasan (2016)
	Preeclampsia and fetal hypotrophy	F. Gilmiyarova, V.Radomskaya
	Iron deficiency anemia	et al. (2007)
	Onychomycosis	Shatohin M., Konoplya A. (2011)
	Chronic generalized periodontitis	Shatohin M., Konoplya A. (2011)
	Helicobacter pylori antibodies in oral fluid	Yanchenko M. (2011)
	Chronic prostatitis	Bektasova M., Kapcov V. (2014)
	The combination of chronic prostatitis with benign	Suslova E., Vasilyeva L. (2012)
	prostatic hyperplasia	Gavrilyuk V. (2011)
	Breast cancer	Doyle B., Quigley J. et al. (2014)
	Tuberculosis	Rizzato C., Campa D. et al.
	Atherosclerosis with complications	(2013)
	Appendicular peritonitis in children	Sadreddini M., Rasmi Y. et al.
	Hemolytic disease of the newborn with A-blood	(2011)
	group mothers	B. Mroczek et al. (2018)
	Pancreatic cancer	D. Stakisaitis (2018)
	Gastroesophageal reflux disease	A. Erden
	Asthma	
	Bladder cancer	
	Mediterranean fever	
B (III)	Pneumonia	Averbah M. (1985)
	Postoperative infection	Dizik G. (1990)
	Osteochondrosis with radicular syndrome	Subbotina T.(2012)
	Sciatica	Shevchenko E. (2010)
	MGTFR mutation	K. Jamamuru (2012)
	Chronic inflammatory processes in women	Shatohin M., Konoplya A. (2011)
	reproductive system	Suslova E., Vasilyeva L. (2013)
	Damage of the coronary artery associated with	Subbotina T., Petuhova A.
	Kawasaki disease	(2012)
	Chronic prostatitis	Stolbova E., Bane B. (2009)
	The combination of chronic obstructive bronchitis	Mortazavi H., Lotfi G. (2015)
	with coronary heart disease	Ramamoorthy B., Varghese S.S.
	Thrombosis	(2015)
	Brain neoplasms	T. T. Lao et al. (2014)
	Gingivitis	
	Periodontal disease	
	HBV	
AB (IV)	Acute respiratory viral infection	L. Grebenshikov (2001),
	Sore throat	S. Garmonov et al. (2006)
	Chronic tonsillitis	Sheng Liming (2013)
	Sinusitis	
	Nasopharynx cancer	

Table 7.
Possibility of pathological process development in ABO blood groups.

ABO blood group

Characteristic	O (I)	A (II)	B (III)	AB (IV)
Protein	N	N	−	+++
Albumin	−	−−−	+++	++
α1	+++	N	−−	N
α2	+++	N	−−	−
β-Globulin	+++	N	−−	−
γ-Globulin	+++	−−−	−−	−
IgA	+++	−−−−	−−−	N
IgG	N	+++	−−−	N
IgM	N	+++	−−−	N
Thymol turbidity test	N	+++	−	−−−−
CRP	+++	N	−−−−	−−
Urea	+++	N	N	−−−−
Uric acid	−−−−	+	N	++
Creatinine	N	N	N	N
Bilirubin	+	−	+	−−−−
ALT	N	N	++	++
AST	−−−−	−	++++	N
GGT	++++	−−−	N	−−
Cholesterol	+	−−−	+++	−−
TAG	+++	++++	−	−−−−
HDL	−−	−−	N	N
LDL	−−	−	−−	++
Lipase	−	−	++	−−−−
Glucose	−−−	−−	++	−−
Lactate dehydrogenase	+++	N	+++	−−−−
Amylase	+++	N	−−−	++

Table 8.
Metabolic characteristic of ABO blood groups (N stands for average results for general population; "+" and "−"—the degree of deviation compared to general population).

The level of hemoglobin in the blood is the lowest, while the saturation of each erythrocyte with hemoglobin is maximum, which ensures full blood transport of gases. A (II) of the second blood group is characterized by the lowest hematocrit value, the average hemoglobin content in one erythrocyte, the average platelet volume, and the maximum indicator of the number of leukocytes, neutrophils, and lymphocytes. Carriers of B (III) blood group showed the largest volume of platelets and the maximum of the average concentration of hemoglobin in one erythrocyte. In persons with AB (IV) blood group, the highest absolute and relative content of lymphocytes, which are the basis of cellular and humoral immunity, is noted. Tendency to lymphocytosis, a higher level of the spectrum of immunoglobulins is an indicator of the intensity of specific resistance and sufficient compensatory reserve in patients with AB (IV) blood group (**Figure 1**).

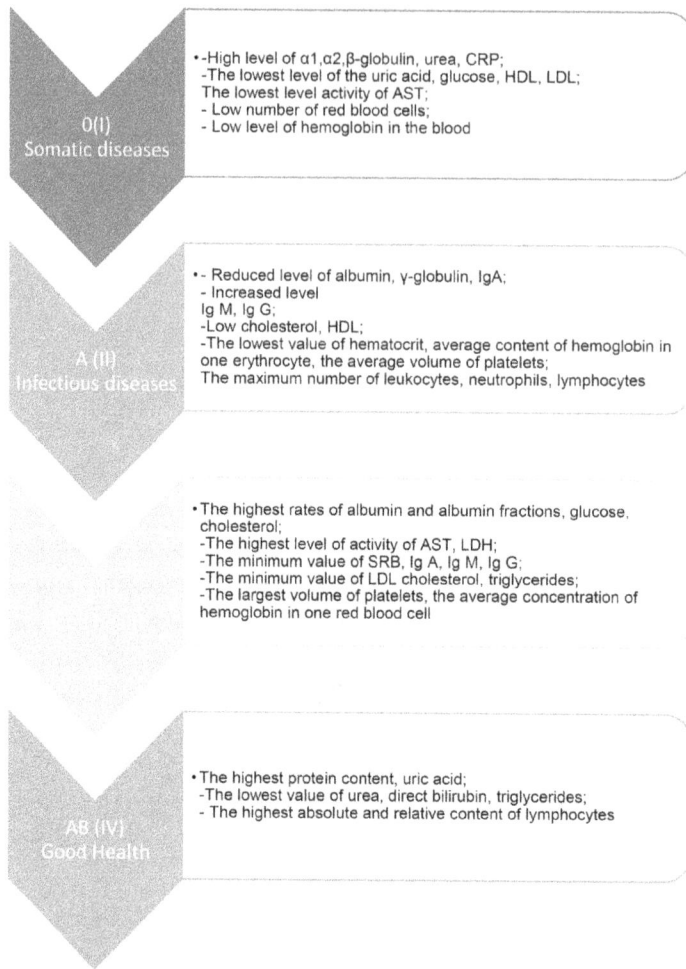

Figure 1.
Biological diversity associated with ABO blood groups.

4. Conclusions

The results obtained in silico by computer prediction with PASS program show that antigens A and B influence on intermolecular processes, protein-protein interaction, maintain balance by regulating protein, carbohydrate, lipid metabolism, antioxidant processes, and tissue respiration quite differently which can be explained with their structure and conformational features.

The series of experiments clearly showed biodiversity in metabolic state of different ABO groups which allow us to create metabolic passport for each blood group summarizing the key data [19].

We found out that the carriers of O (I) blood group suffer from somatic diseases more recently than the other blood group carriers, while the carriers of A blood group are predisposed for infectious diseases, and the carriers B (III) and AB (IV) blood groups are more likely to show metabolic stability.

To summarize, methods of molecular modeling and forecasting allow us to broaden the fundamental knowledge about the molecules' properties and to successfully predict new possible biological effects, as well as molecular mechanisms for its realization in complex interactions of ligands and their targets.

Acknowledgements

The authors appreciate the help and support of the head of Samara State Medical University, professor G.P. Kotelnikov. Our work is dedicated to the 100th anniversary of Samara State Medical University.

Conflict of interest

The authors state that they have no conflicts of interest.

Thanks

The authors thank the chair of Fundamental and Clinical Biochemistry with laboratory diagnostic of Samara State Medical University.

Author details

Frida N. Gylmiyarova[1*], Elena Ryskina[2], Nataliya Kolotyeva[1], Valeriia Kuzmicheva[1] and Oksana Gusyakova[1]

1 Samara State Medical University, Samara, Russia

2 Peoples' Friendship University of Russia, Moscow, Russia

*Address all correspondence to: bio-sam@yandex.ru

IntechOpen

References

[1] Franchini M, Bonfanti C. Evolutionary aspects of ABO blood group in humans. Clinica Chimica Acta. 2015;**444**:66-71

[2] Franchini M, Liumbruno G. ABO blood group: Old dogma, new perspectives. Clinical Chemistry and Laboratory Medicine. 2013;**51**(8):1545-1553

[3] Gylmiyarova F, Ryskina E, Kolotieva N, Potekhina V, Gorbacheva I. Protein-ligand interactions: The influence of minor components of metabolism. Siberian Medical Review. 2017;(6):12-21

[4] Kastritis P, Bonvin A. On the binding affinity of macromolecular interactions: Daring to ask why proteins interact. Journal of the Royal Society Interface. 2012;**10**(79):20120835

[5] Muronetz V, Barinova K, Stroylova Y, Semenyuk P, Schmalhausen E. Glyceraldehyde-3-phosphate dehydrogenase: Aggregation mechanisms and impact on amyloid neurodegenerative diseases. International Journal of Biological Macromolecules. 2017;**100**:55-66

[6] Stepanchikova AV, Lagunin AA, Filimonov DA, Poroikov VV. Prediction of biological activity spectra for substances: Evaluation on the diverse set of drugs-like structures. Current Medicinal Chemistry. 2003;**10**:225-233

[7] Poroikov VV, Akimov D, Shabelnikova E, Filimonov D. Top 200 medicines: Can new actions be discovered through computer-aided prediction? SAR and QSAR in Environmental Research. 2001;**12**(4):327-344

[8] Rios M, Bianca C. The role of blood group antigens in infectious diseases. Seminars in Hematology. 2000;**37**(2):177-185

[9] Daniels G, Fletcher A, Garratty G, Henry S, Jorgensen J, Judd W, et al. Blood group terminology 2004: From the International Society of Blood Transfusion committee terminology for red cell surface antigens. Vox Sanguinis. 2004;**87**(4):304-316

[10] Risch H, Lu L, Wang J, Zhang W, Ni Q, Gao Y, et al. ABO blood group and risk of pancreatic cancer: A study in Shanghai and meta-analysis. American Journal of Epidemiology. 2013;**177**(12):1326-1337

[11] Malecki M, Kolsut P, Proczka R. Angiogenic and antiangiogenic gene therapy. Gene Therapy. 2005;**12**(S1):S159-S169

[12] Bell R, Rube H, Kreig A, Mancini A, Fouse S, Nagarajan R, et al. Abstract B12: GABP selectively binds and activates the mutant TERT promoter across multiple cancer types. Cancer Research. 2015;**75**(23 Supplement):B12-B12

[13] Kato K, Ishiwa A. The role of carbohydrates in infection strategies of enteric pathogens. Tropical Medicine and Health. 2015;**43**(1):41-52

[14] Gao J, He H, Jiang W, Chang X, Zhu L, Luo F, et al. Salidroside ameliorates cognitive impairment in a D-galactose-induced rat model of Alzheimer's disease. Behavioural Brain Research. 2015;**293**:27-33

[15] Cristina Stanca-Kaposta E, Gamblin D, Screen J, Liu B, Snoek L, Davis B, et al. Carbohydrate molecular recognition: A spectroscopic investigation of carbohydrate-aromatic interactions. Physical Chemistry Chemical Physics. 2007;**9**(32):4444

[16] Milland EY, Xing PX, McKenzie FC, et al. Carbohydrate residues downstream of the terminal Galα(1, 3)

Gal epitope modulate the specificity of xenoreactive antibodies. Immunology and Cell Biology. 2007;**85**:623-632

[17] Agostino M, Sandrin M, Thompson P, Yuriev E, Ramsland P. Identification of preferred carbohydrate binding modes in xenoreactive antibodies by combining conformational filters and binding site maps. Glycobiology. 2010;**20**(6):724-735

[18] Gylmiyarova F, Radomskaya N, Gergel N, Kotelknikov G, editors. Blood Groups: Biological Variability of Cellular Metabolism in Norm and Pathology. Moscow: Izvestiya; 2007

[19] Gylmiyarova F, Kolotyeva N, Potekhina V, Baisheva G, Ryskina E. The lactate role in intramolecular regulation of proteins interaction. Meditsinskiy Al'manakh. 2017;**2**(47):99-101

www.ingramcontent.com/pod-product-compliance
Lightning Source LLC
Chambersburg PA
CBHW081239190326
41458CB00016B/5845